Peter St George-Hyslop, University of Toronto, Toronto (Canada)
Robert Terry, University of California, La Jolla (USA)
Henry Wisniewski, Institute for Basic Research in Development Disabilities, Staten Island (USA)
Edouard Zarifian, Centre Hospitalier Universitaire, Caen (France)

F. Boller F. Forette Z. Khachaturian
M. Poncet Y. Christen (Eds.)

Heterogeneity of Alzheimer's Disease

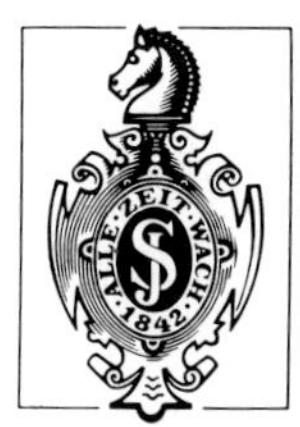

Springer-Verlag
Berlin Heidelberg New York
London Paris Tokyo Hong Kong
Barcelona Budapest

Boller, Francois, Prof. Dr.
INSERM U324, 2ter rue de Alesia
F-75015 Paris

Forette, F.
Hopital Broca
54 rue Pascal
F-75013 Paris

Khachaturian, Z.S.
National Institute on Aging
National Institutes of Health
Bethesda, MD 20892, USA

Poncet, Michel
Clinique de Neurologie, CHU La Timone
Bd Jean Moulin,
F-13385 Marseille Cedex 05

Christen, Yves, PH. D.
Fondation Ipsen pour La Recherche Therapeutique
30, rue Cambronne
F-75737 Paris CEDEX 15

ISBN 3-540-55918-3 Springer-Verlag Berlin Heidelberg New York
ISBN 0-387-55918-3 Springer-Verlag New York Berlin Heidelberg

Typesetting: Cicero Lasersatz, 8900 Augsburg
Printed: Druckhaus Beltz, 6944 Hemsbach
Bookbinding: J. Schäffer, 6718 Grünstadt
27/3145/5 4 3 2 1 0 – Printed on acid-free paper

Preface

This volume contains the proceedings of a symposium held in Marseille on April 6, 1992, on the topic "Heterogeneity of Alzheimer's disease." This was the eighth of a continuing and very successful series of meetings related to Alzheimer's disease organized by the Fondation Ipsen pour la Recherche Thérapeutique. These symposia, known as "Colloques médecine et recherche," started in 1987 and have dealt with widely different aspects of the disease such as *immunology, genetics, neuronal grafting, biological markers, imaging, growth factors,* and last year's less conventional topic of *Neurophilosophy and Alzheimer's disease.* The next IPSEN symposium dedicatet to Alzheimer's disease will take place in Lyon on June 21, 1993, and will deal with *"Amyloid protein precursors in development, aging, and alzheimer's disease."* It is being organized by Konrad Beyreuther, Colin Masters, Marc Trillet, and Yves Christen.

Until a few years ago, several names were used to refer to the most common cause of dementia in the elderly. They included such terms as "senile psychosis," "organic brain syndrome," and "senile dementia." Following Kraepelin, the term "Alzheimer's disease" was often restricted to an uncommon condition starting at a younger age (before 60 or 65 years of age). In 1978, the conclusions of a symposium organized by Robert Katzman, Robert Terry, and Katherine Bick pointed out that there was an "increasing recognition that the clinical and pathological manifestations are almost identical in the presenium and in the senium." This and the success in the United States of the Alzheimer Disease and Related Disorders Association (ADRDA, now called Alzheimer Association) were among the factors contributing to the much more widespread use of the term "Alzheimer's disease" in recent years.

Independently of the nomenclature, it has always been obvious to anyone dealing with demented patients that there are marked differences among patients. In fact, once we start taking a close look, we find that cases always differ from one another and that no patient is ever exactly like any other. Does this symply reflect the variability found in any disease, or does it represent the expression of different pathological phenomena?

This symposium gathered researchers with backgrounds as different as epidemiology, clinical neurology and geriatrics, neuropsychology, neuropathology, molecular biology, and genetics. The primary purpose of the meeting was to provide elements that might allow a rational answer to the question of heterogeneity of Alzheimer's disease. This question is of great theoretical interest, but with the appearance of new therapeutic interventions, it may well start having a very significant practical importance.

The city of Marseille and its neighbor Aix-en-Provence have a long-standing tradition of academic excellence in many fields including neurology and neurosciences and we are indebted to the Mayor of Aix, Dr Jean-Francois Picheral, who provided a very warm welcome to the participants. Once again, the organization of the meeting was perfect in all respects, thanks to the efforts of Mrs. Jacqueline Mervaillie and her colleagues. We also wish to thank the contributors to this volume, the authors of posters, and all the participants to the meeting. Our particular gratitude goes to Dr. Zaven Khatchaturian who in the past several years has significantly contributed to the development of research on Alzheimer's disease in the United States and other countries. Our thanks also go to Professor Michel Poncet and Profesor George Serratrice who kindly acted as session chairs, and to Mary Lynn Gage who provided editorial assistance.

François Boller
Yves Christen

Contents

Contributors

Alberts, M.
  Joseph and Kathleen Bryan Alzheimer's Disease Research Center,
  Duke University Medical Center, Durham, MC 27710, USA

Amaducci, L.
  Department of Neurologic and Psychiatric Sciences, University of Florence,
  Viale Morgagni 85, 50134 Florence, Italy

Béland, R.
  Laboratoire Théophile-Alajouanine, C. H. Côte-des-Neiges,
  4565, chemin de la Reine-Marie, Montréal, Québec H3W 1W5, Canada

Bert, P.
  Hôpital Broca, 54 rue Pascal, 75013 Paris, France

Bhasin, R.
  Department of Psychiatry, State University of New York at Stony Brook,
  Stony Brook, NY 11794–8101, USA

Bird, T. D.
  Departments of Medicine and Pathology, University of Washington Medical
  School and the VA Medical Center, Seattle, WA 98018, USA

Boller, F.
  INSERM U324, 2 ter rue d'Alexia, 75014 Paris, France

Breuil, V.
  Hôpital Broca, 54 rue Pascal, 75013 Paris, France

Bruni, A.
  SMID-SUD, Scala 4, via dei Campione,
  Lamezzia Terme, CZ, Italy

Buxbaum, J. D.
  Laboratory of Molecular and Cellular Neuroscience,
  The Rockefeller University,
  1230 York Avenue, New York, NQ 10021, USA

Caporaso, G. L.
Laboratory of Molecular and Cellular Neuroscience,
The Rockefeller University,
1230 York Avenue, New York, NY 10021, USA

Chui, H. C.
University of Southern California School of Medicine, Los Angeles
and Geriatric Neurobehavior and Alzheimer Center, 12838 Erickson Street,
Downey, CA 90242, USA

Crapper McLachlan, D. R.
Department of Medicine, Centre for Research in Neurodegenerative
Disease, Tanz Neuroscience Building, Univesity of Toronto,
Ontario M5S1A8, Canada

Crystal, H. A.
Albert Einstein College of Medicine, 1300 Morris Park Avenue, Bronx,
NY 10461, USA

Czernik, A. J.
Laboratory of Molecular and Cellular Neuroscience, The Rockefeller
University, 1230 York Avenue, New York, NY 10021, USA

Davies, P.
Albert Einstein College of Medicine, 1300 Morris Park Avenue, Bronx,
NY 10461, USA

Delacourte, A.
INSERM U 156, Place de Verdun, 59045 Lille CEDEX, France

Delaère, P.
Laboratoire de Neuropathologie R. Escourolle, Hôpital de la Salpêtrière,
47, Boulevard de l'Hôpital, 75651 Parix CEDEX 13, France

Dickson, D. W.
Albert Einstein College of Medicine, 1300 Morris Park Avenue, Bronx,
NY 10461, USA

Duyckaerts, C.
Laboratoire de Neuropathologie R. Escourolle, Hôpital de la Salpêtrière,
47, Boulevard de l'Hôpital, 75651 Paris CEDEX 13, France

Fink, J.
Department of Neurology, University of Michigan Medical Center,
Ann Arbor, MI 48104, USA

Foncin, J-F.
Laboratoire de Neurohistologie, Ecole Pratique des Hautes Etudes,
Hôpital de la Salpêtrière, 75651 Paris CEDEX 13, France

Forette, F.
Hôpital Broca, 54 rue Pascal, 75013 Paris, France

Frigard, B.
INSERM U 156, Place de Verdun, 59045 Lille CEDEX, France

Gandy, S. E.
Laboratory of Molecular and Cellular Neuroscience, The Rockefeller
University, 1230 York Avenue, New York, NY 10021, USA

Gilbert, J.
Joseph and Kathleen Bryan Alzheimer's Disease Research Center,
Duke University Medical Center, Durham, MC 27710, USA

Goldgaber, D.
Department of Psychiatry, State University of New York at Stony Brook,
Stony Brook, NY 11794–8101, USA

Grafman, J.
Cognitive Neuroscience Section, Medical Neurology Branch, National
Institute of Neurological Disorders and Stroke, Bethesda, MD 20892, USA

Greengard, P.
Laboratory of Molecular and Cellular Neuroscience, The Rockefeller
University, 1230 York Avenue, New York, NY 10021, USA

Haines, J. L.
Molecular Neurogentics Laboratory, Massachusetts General Hospital,
Bldg 149, 13th Street, Charlestown, MA 02129, USA

Hardy J.
Alzheimer's Disease Research Group, Department of Biochemistry,
St Mary's Hospital Medical School, London, W2 1PG, UK and Suncoast
Dementia Research Group, Department of Psychiatry, University of South
Florida, Tampa FL 33612 (USA)

Hauw, J.-J.
Laboratoire de Neuropathologie R. Escourolle, Hôpital de la Salpêtrière,
47, Boulevard de l'Hôpital, 75651 Paris CEDEX 13, France

Iverfeldt, K.
Laboratory of Molecular and Cellular Neuroscience, The Rockefeller
University, 1230 York Avenue, New York, NY 10021, USA

Joanette, Y.
Laboratoire Theôphile-Alajouanine, C. H. Côte-des-Neiges, 4565,
chemin de la Reine-Marie, Montréal, Québec H3W 1W5, Canada

Kennedy, A. M.
Department of Neurology, St. Mary's Hospital, Praed Street, London W2, UK

Khachaturian, Z. S.
  National Institute on Aging, National Institutes of Health, Bethesda,
  MD 20892, USA

Lippi, A.
  Department of Neurologic and Psychiatric Sciences, University of Florence,
  Viale Morgagni 85, 50134 Florence, Italy

Lukiw, W.
  Department of Medicine, Centre for Research in Neurodegenerative
  Disease, Tanz Neuroscience Building, University of Toronto,
  Ontario
  M5S1A8, Canada

Lyness, S.
  University of Southern California, School of Medicine, Los Angeles, CA,
  USA

Matthiace, L. A.
  Albert Einstein College of Medicine, 1300 Morris Park Avenue, Bronx,
  NY 10461, USA

Mayeux, R.
  Columbia University, College of Physicians and Surgeons, The Memory
  Disorders Clinic of the New York State Psychiatric Institute and the Center
  for Alzheimer's Disease Research in the City of New York and The
  Gertrude H. Sergievsky Center, 630 West 168th St., New York,
  NY 10032, USA

Mesulam, M-M.
  Department of Neurology Beth Israel Hospital, 3300 Brookline Avenue,
  Boston, MA 02215, USA

Montesi, M. P.
  SMID-SUD, Scala 4, via dei Campione, Lamezzia Terme, CZ, Italy

Mortilla, M.
  Department of Medicine, Centre for Research in Neurodegenerative
  Disease, Tanz Neuroscience Building, University of Toronto,
  Ontario, M5S1A8, Canada

Nairn, A. C.
  Laboratory of Molecular and Cellular Neuroscience, The Rockefeller
  University, 1230 York Avenue, New York, NY 10021, USA

Nemens, E.M.
  Departments of Medicine and Pathology, University of Washington Medical
  School and the VA Medical Center, Seattle, WA 98108, USA

Newman, S. K.
Department of Neurology, St Mary's Hospital, Praed Street, London W2, UK

Nochlin, D.
Departments of Medicine and Pathology, University of Washington Medical
School and the VA Medical Center, Seattle, WA 98108, USA

Norderstedt, C.
Laboratory of Molecular and Cellular Neuroscience,
The Rockefeller University, 1230 York Avenue, New York, NY 10021, USA

Peacock, M.
Department of Neurology, University of Michigan Medical Center,
Ann Arbor, MI 48104, USA

Pericak-Vance, M.
Joseph and Kathleen Bryan Alzheimer's Disease Research Center,
Duke University Medical Center, Durham, MC 27710, USA

Pinessi, L.
Department of Neurology, University of Turin, via Chereasco, Turin, Italy

Poissant, A.
Laboratoire Theóphile-Alajouanine, C. H. Côte-des-Neiges, 4565,
chemin de la Reine-Marie, Montréal, Québec H3W 1W5, Canada

Polinsky, R. J.
Sandoz Research Institute, Sandoz Pharmaceuticals Inc., Hannover,
New Jersey, USA

Pollen, D.
Department of Neurology, University of Massachusetts Medical Center,
55 Lake Avenue North, Worcester, MA 01605, USA

Rainero, I.
Department of Neurology, University of Turin, via Cherasco, Turin, Italy

Ramabhadran, T. V.
Laboratory of Molecular and Cellular Neuroscience, The Rockefeller
University 1230 York Avenue, New York, NY 10021, USA

Rogaev, E.
Department of Medicine, Centre for Research in Neurodegenerative
Disease, Tanz Neuroscience Building, University of Toronto,
Ontario, M5S1A8, Canada

Roses, A.
Joseph and Kathleen Bryan Alzheimer's Disease Research Center,
Duke University Medical Center, Durham, MC 27710, USA

Rossor, M. N.
Department of Neurology, St. Mary's Hospital, Praed Street, London W2, UK

Sano, M.
Columbia University, College of Physicians and Surgeons, The Memory
Disorders Clinic of the New York State Psychiatric Instituts and the Center for
Alzheimer's Disease Research in the City of New York, 168th Street,
New York, NY 10032, USA

Saunders, A.
Joseph and Kathleen Bryan Alzheimer's Disease Research Center,
Duke University Medical Center, Durham, MC 27710, USA

Schellenberg, G. D.
Departments of Medicine and Pathology, University of Washington Medical
School and the VA Medical Center, Seattle, WA 98108, USA

Schneider, L. S.
University of Southern California, School of Medicine, Los Angeles, CA, USA

Schwartzbach, C.
Joseph and Kathleen Bryan Alzheimer's Disease Research Center,
Duke University Medical Center, Durham, MC 27710, USA

Ska, B.
Laboratoire Theôphile-Alajouanine, C. H. Côte-des-Neiges, 4565,
chemin de la Reine-Marie, Montréal, Québe H3W 1W5, Canada

Sobel, E.
University of Southern California, School of Medicine, Los Angeles, CA, USA

Sorbi, S.
Department of Neurology, University of Florence, Viale Morgagni, Florence,
Italy

St George-Hyslop, P. H.
Department of Medicine, Centre for Research in Neurodegenerative
Disease, Tanz Neuroscience Building, University of Toronto, Ontario,
M5S1A8, Canada

Stern, Y.
The Gertrude H. Sergievsky Center, 630 West 168th St., New York,
NY 10032, USA

Sumi, S. M.
Departments of Medicine and Pathology, University of Washington Medical
School and the VA Medical Center, Seattle, WA 98108, USA

Suzuki, T.
   Laboratory of Molecular and Cellular Neuroscience, The Rockefeller
   University, 1230 York Avenue, New York, NY 10021, USA

Tanzi, R.
   Molecular Neurogenetics Laboratory, Massachusetts General Hospital,
   Bldg 149, 13th Street, Charlestown, MA 02129, USA

Taylor, H.
   Joseph and Kathleen Bryan Alzheimer's Disease Research Center,
   Duke University Medical Center, Durham, MC 27710, USA

Tupler, R.
   Department of Medicine, Centre for Research in Neurodegenerative
   Disease, Tanz Neuroscience Building, University of Toronto,
   Ontario, M5S1A8, Canada

Vaula, G.
   Department of Medicine, Centre for Research in Neurodegenerative
   Disease, Tanz Neuroscience Building, University of Toronto,
   Ontario, M5S1A8, Canada

Vermersch, P.
   INSERM U 156, Place de Verdun, 59045 Lille CEDEX, France

Wattez, A.
   INSERM U 156, Place de Verdun, 59045 Lille CEDEX, France

Weintraub, S.
   Department of Neurology Beth Israel Hospital, 330 Brookline Avenue,
   Boston, MA 02215, USA

Wijsman, E. M.
   Departments of Medicine and Pathology, University of Washington Medical
   School and the VA Medical Center, Seattle, WA 98108, USA

Wu, E.
   Albert Einstein College of Medicine, 1300 Morris Park Avenue, Bronx,
   NY 10461, USA

Yen-S-H.C.
   Albert Einstein College of Medicine, 1300 Morris Park Avenue, Bronx,
   NY 10461, USA

An Overview of Scientific Issues Associated with the Heterogeneity of Alzheimer's Disease

Z. S. Khachaturian

At present no scientist can say with assurance whether Alzheimer's disease (AD) is a single disease, a complex syndrome, with many subtypes and varieties of patterns in its manifestations, or many different diseases with similar clusters of symptoms. The heterogeneity of the disease is demonstrated in many of its aspects: age of onset, duration, clinical course, types and patterns of neurological and psychiatric symptoms, response to treatment and neuropathological lesions.

A number of the scientific problems facing the field of AD research are directly associated with heterogeneity in the expression of this disease. Although during the last 14 years significant progress has been made in identifiying and describing the different manifestations of AD, the underlying biological mechanisms of the heterogeneity still remain to be uncovered. The general problem of heterogeneity provides an unusually rich array of scientific opportunities for further research direction. The following is a brief discussion of some these research avenues that need further investigation.

Biological Basis of Heterogeneity

The search for genes associated with various brain metabolic dysfunctions and abnormal processing of cytoskeletal proteins promises to be one of the most productive lines of research in uncovering the cause(s) of this disease. The recent findings of mutations in the APP gene have created great excitement and given special impetus to the search for other loci and other mutations. Unfortunately, identifying the locus and the nature of the mutation will not be sufficient; this field still needs to determine the functional consequences of these genetic changes and how they affect protein synthesis or alter metabolic activity.

Presently it is not clear whether mutations in genes are a necessary and sufficient condition to cause the disease or whether one or more additional biological insult(s) are necessary to trigger the degenerative processes of AD. If there is a relationship between genetic predisposition for AD and environmental factors or other systemic metabolic dysfunctions, the mechanism for the interaction between genes and such triggering factors is not well studied. The field needs to know how changes in metabolic functions, the immune system,

F. Boller et al. (Eds.)
Heterogeneity of Alzheimer's Disease
© Springer-Verlag Berlin Heidelberg 1992

neuroendocrine factors, infectious agents, and exposure to toxins influence the expression of the disease or modulate its course.

There is also a need for further investigation of co-morbidity with AD of other neurodegenerative diseases and systemic disorders. The patient's health history, dietary habits, occupation, exposure to toxins and life experiences, such as education, need to be studied more systematically. Recent epidemiological investigations have suggested that lack of education might be a risk factor for AD. If these observations are confirmed, they may provide clues to possible mechanisms of heterogeneity by linking risk factors like life experiences to changes in the brain such as synaptic density or synaptic reserve.

Clinical Studies of Heterogeneity

Early in the history of AD research, there were no commonly accepted diagnostic criteria or standardized assessment instruments. Since the mid-1980s, diagnostic criteria have been established and several multicenter collaborative studies initiated to develop, validate, and standardize diagnostic tests. Now the field of clinical research on AD needs to expand its efforts to refine the established criteria. It is time to begin developing a comprehensive diagnostic classification schema that will categorize patients into more homogeneous groups on the basis of clusters of symptoms which are clinically meaningful for treatment or management.

Infrastructure and Resources for Clinical Studies of Heterogeneity

Presently there are very few facilities that are adequate for the conduct of systematic longitudinal studies of the clinical course of AD. The lack of suitable facilities for clinical research, the insidious onset of the disease, its slow progress, and the high cost of research have all contributed to the difficulty of conducting the much-needed longitudinal clinical studies on AD. Yet, to study systematically the problem of heterogeneity in AD, the filed needs longitudinal studies with large numbers of subjects recruited from diverse backgrounds.

Such studies should be designed as collaborative efforts among many centers around the world that are prepared to obtain detailed medical histories and to collect carefully repeated observations on the clinical course of the disease using validated and standardized instruments, tests or observation techniques. These studies should follow the clinical course of the disease from its earliest possible stages through autopsy. It is only through such carefully and methodically conducted studies that it will be possible to establish the clinical pathological correlations of this disease and to begin sorting out answers on the heterogeneity of AD.

In summary, defining the scientific issues related to the heterogeneity of AD is critical to realizing advancement in our knowledge of this devastating disease. The topic of heterogeneity is important from the perspectives of what scientists need to know; better understanding of the biological basis of heterogeneity should provide new insights into possible etiologic factors and lead to refinement of theories on the biology of dementing process(es). The topic is also important from the perspective of clinical care because, undoubtedly, better knowledge of heterogeneity would lead to improvements in the design of clinical trials and the development of specifically targeted treatment strategies. Finally, more information of heterogeneity should lead to the development of well-conceived patient care and management approaches, thus improving the quality of life for both the patient and care provider.

In closing, I want to express my deep appreciation to the Foundation IPSEN for having the foresight to organize this symposium on timely topics concerning Alzheimer's disease. I am particularly grateful to Jacqueline Mervaillie and Yves Christen for their efforts to include me as a participant in this important conference.

A Comparison of Clinical Outcome and Survival in Various Forms of Alzheimer's Disease

R. Mayeux, Y. Stern, and *M. Sano*

Summary

The heterogeneous character of Alzheimer's disease (AD) has significant etiologic and clinical implications. Heterogeneity makes the definition of AD less than precise, and it has made it difficult to establish a single etiology, be it genetic or environmental. For example, the aphasic "subtypes" of AD have been associated with an increased likelihood of having family history of dementia in a first-degree relative (Breitner and Folstein, 1984; Breitner et al., 1986). A different phenotype, characterized by early onset AD with myoclonus and seizures, was found to exhibit linkage to chromosome 21 (St George-Hyslop et al., 1987). Not all patients with familial AD manifest aphasia; neither does this imply specificity to a particular etiology.

Clinical heterogeneity could also reflect pleiotrophy (a single gene with multiple effects or manifestations). Similarly, a series of studies has established that a proportion of patients with AD develop extrapyramidal signs, mycolonus or psychosis The appearance of these signs might predict the rate of disease progression in terms of both intellectual deterioration, functional decline and death. The cumulative risk of developing extrapyramidal signs or psychosis is highest in early stages of AD, while the risk of myoclonus occurs later. For patients with AD the risk of dying is also significantly increased once myoclonus or extrapyramidal signs appear. It has now been implied that this clinical heterogeneity does not define "clinical subtypes" of AD; rather these signs appear to be development manifestations that reflect disease progression and, presumably, the underlying pathophysiology and etiology.

Phenotypic Variation:
Clinical Heterogeneity in Alzheimer's Disease

Family studies have shown that a "young onset" phenotype is consistently "linked" to chromosome 21 (St George-Hylops et al., 1987, 1990). Moreover, there is evidence that a specific point mutation in codon 717 of the APP gene on chromosome 21 (APP_{717}) is present in affected members, and not in unaffected members, of five unrelated families with the young onset phenotype (Goate et al., 1991; Naruse et al., 1991; Lucotte et al., 1991; Murrell et al., 1991; Chartier-Harlin et al., 1991).

F. Boller et al. (Eds.)
Heterogeneity of Alzheimer's Disease
© Springer-Verlag Berlin Heidelberg 1992

Other clinical and pathological data sustain the view that this phenotype may be unique. Duffy et al. (1988) reported "spongy" change in the neocortex of patients with young onset familial AD. The syndrome associated with this form of AD also included myoclonic jerks, aphasia progressing to complete mutism and a rapid progression of illness leading to death. Similary, Bird et al. (1983) reported that patients with familial AD and myoclonus often had the greatest reduction in choline acetyltransferase activity in the brain at the time of post-mortem examination. Less consistent has been the observation that there is a reduction in the cerebrospinal fluid content of the major metabolites of serotonin and dopamine in patients with myoclonus (Kaye et al., 1988a, b). However, neither report related these finding to a genetic or environmental etiology.

An aphasic form of AD has also been suggested as a specific "subtype" and proposed as a specific phenotype with a genetic etiology. The observation that a disturbance in language was the major defining feature was first mentioned by Breitner and Folstein (1984) when they noted that patients with familial AD were unable to complete a sentence task from the Mini-Mental State Examination. Moreover, affected first-degree family members were similarly agraphic. In fact, an extended battery of tests examining for aphasia, agraphia and apraxia found a significantly higher frequency of language disturbance in the relatives of "agraphic" patients with AD than among sporadic cases. Breitner et al. (1986) found that the life time (to age 90) risk of dementia in first-degree relatives of probands with the "agraphic" form of AD was approximately 50%, suggesting an autosomal dominant gene with age-dependent penetrance.

Seltzer and Sherwin (1983) also found that men with onset of AD before age 65 were more likely to show language impairment, particularly diminished spontaneous speech, verbal comprehension, confrontation naming and impaired writing. Life expectancy was also reduced for these individuals. Their explanation of these finding implicated a genetic vulnerability in the left hemisphere which was affected in AD.

Jorm (1985) has offered an alternative explanation for these observations, suggesting that the cross-sectional nature of these studies did not exclude the possibility that these "subtypes" simply represent different stages of the disease. That would mean that all patients with AD, regardless of their etiology, might eventually develop aphasia. Jorm (1985) pointed out that data presented by both groups of authors indicated diminished survival for the language disordered groups. In addition, others have noted a relationship between language impairment and survival (Heyman et al., 1983).

Thus the alternative explanation for phenotypic variations or clinical heterogeneity is that they represent various stages of the disease and not a specific phenotype associated with a particular genotype or etiology. Perhaps the only exception is the young onset AD phenotype associated with the familial AD (FAD) gene on chromosome 21 (St George-Hyslop et al., 1987, 1990).

While it may be critical to separate each individual syndrome or clinical variant within the diagnosis of AD, this leads to the assumption that various clinical features characterize specific etiologies. Thus far the only consistent clinical feature associated with the FAD genotype (chromosome 21) is a young age at disease onset. Seizures, myoclonus, mutism and rapid progression are inconsistent features, and it should be noted that not all young onset forms of AD are familial. Further, the linkage to chromosome 19 in familial AD with onset in later life was not associated with a particular phenotype (Pericak-Vance et al., 1991).

Clinical heterogeneity and the natural history of Alzheimer's disease

Although clinical heterogeneity has been recognized for several years in patients with AD, two reports in 1985 (Mayeux et al., 1985; Chui et al., 1985) clearly indicated that heterogeneity might be considered an important factor in disease progression.The major clinical signs that have been associated with more rapid progression are described below.

1. Extrapyramidal signs: characterized by rigidity (resistance to passive movement of the arms and legs) bradykinesia (slowness of movement). Occasionally, extrapyramidal signs are the result of dopamine blockade from phenothiazine administration: Excluding these patients, howewer, we (Mayeux et al., 1985) and others (Chui et al., 1985) noted that the "extrapyramidal" form of AD seemed to be accompanied by more rapid progression of disease. Nearly 30% of patients in a cross-sectional study were found to have the signs which we felt were unrelated to disease duration.
2. Myoclonic jerks: characterized by brief, irregular muscle jerks; found to be present in 5% to 10% of the patients with AD. Most descriptions indicate that patients with myoclonus are younger than others at the time of disease onset but, as will become apparent, myoclonus may occur as a late manifestation of AD as well. Myoclonus and extrapyramidal signs coexisted in a small number of patients.

The work of Chui et al. (1985) supported the view that disease progression was much more rapid in patients with these signs, although both of these studies were cross-sectional, making it difficult to appreciate the longitudinal nature of these observations.

Both clinical and pathological data supported the unique nature of these observations. Ditter and Mirra (1987) reported depigmentation in the substantia nigra and the presence of subcortical Lewy body formation in patients with the "extrapyramidal" form of AD. Duffy et al. (1988) described "spongy change" in the outher layers of the cerebral cortex associated with a familial form of AD with myclonus and mutism. Kaye et al. (1988a, b) described reduced concentrations of the major metabolites, serotonin and dopamine in both of these syndromes.

Whether these manifestations of AD represented a "subgroup or subtype" was less important than establishing the usefulness of these signs as predictive features. In two longitudinal studies (Stern et al. 1987, 1990) of the same patients we attempted to determine the time period from first assessment to a point at which impairment in cognitive function or activities of daily living was reached. We covaried by the presence of myoclonus, extrapyramidal signs and psychosis to examine these endpoints. Using survival analysis to examine the rate of disease progression, we found that patients with extrapyramidal signs reached and advanced stage of dementia more rapidly than equally demented patients without these clinical signs. However, we found no difference in the performance of activities of daily living in these two groups over time. Similar observations were noted for patients who developed psychosis during the disease course, but we could not address myoclonus because so few patients presented with this sign.

As a follow-up to the work of Jorm (1985), we wanted to explore the possibility that these clinical signs represent developmental stages of AD that reflect disease progression rather than clinical signs that predict disease severity. To examine this, we again (Chen et al., 1991) returned to our original cohort. The patients had been followed consistently for nearly five years at six-month intervals, and all deaths in which an autopsy was performed confirmed AD.

We used the Kaplan-Meier survival analysis to estimate the cumulative risks of developing the clinical signs during the course of illness. We determined the percentage of individuals with any of the clinical signs (prevalence of myoclonus, extrapyramidal signs or psychosis) as well as the number of patients who developed these signs (incidence rate of myoclonus, extrapyramidal signs or psychosis) over the follow-up period. The cumulative risk for developing either extrapyramidal signs or psychosis was similar. Both were greater than the cumulative risk of developing myoclonus. However, with disease progression, the probability of developing mycolonus became as great as that of developing the other signs. The assessment allowed us to assume independence among the cumulative risks and suggested that, whereas extrapyramidal signs and psychosis occurred within the first few years of disease, the emergence of myoclonus was a late phenomenon. We used binomial tests, adjusted for multiple comparisons, and found that extrapyramidal signs occurred before myoclonus in 30 of 43 patients, as did psychosis (both $p < 0.05$). Extrapyramidal signs and psychosis were present in equal proportions, 25–28%. The prevalence of myoclonus initially was low (6.9%). However, the incidence or the occurrence of new signs was highest for myoclonus, with 34.3% of the patients developing this sign by their last visit (on average about 7 years). The rates for developing extrapyramidal signs or psychosis were similar, 32.7% and 29.1%, respectively.

These observations led us to develop a different perspective on extrapyramidal signs, psychosis, and myoclonus as well as clinical heterogeneity in general. We began to view them as indicative of disease stages rather than predictors of disease progression. In fact, it is likely that many patients with AD develop extrapyramidal signs early in the disease and that they remain present for a long period. The frequency of myoclonus (less than 7%) was similar to that reported by Chui et al. (1985) in their cross-sectional study, but the relatively high cumulative risk of myoclonus over time suggests that myoclonus is not as uncommon as previously considered. However, because the duration of AD decreases after the appearance of myoclonus, the overall prevalence at any one time in a cross-sectional study would be lower. This phenomenon is the result of the known relationship between prevalence and incidence. (Prevalence equals the product of incidence rate x duration.)

Thus, extrapyramidal signs, psychosis and myoclonus probably represent development stages of AD rather than clinical subtypes or unique phenotypes. The "subtype" or "subgroup" concept of heterogeneity would allow one to view development myoclonus as a distinct subgroup which differs pathologically and perhaps also etiologically from those who develop extrapyramidal signs or psychosis. This concept implies mutual exclusiveness as a subtype. However, it is clear from our data that patients may develop more than one sign and that myoclonus, psychosis and extrapyramidal signs can coexist. Moreover, it suggests that nearly every patient will eventually develop myoclonus but the risk differs during the course of disease.

The probabilistic view implies that clinical signs such as extrapyramidal signs, psychosis and myoclonus, specific levels of function or cognitive deterioration, or even death are disease markers or outcomes and represent different stages of the disease. Patients are somewhat "biologically unique", and it would be reasonable to expect some degree of variability. In fact, the probabilistic view allows one to also interpret the emergence of these signs as landmarks by which to measure disease progression; that is, that once the signs emerge, the survival can be estimated by probability. The advantage of this view is that each disease feature is allowed to emerge with different probabilities at different times and the relationship to other disease features can be properly assessed. This would help determine the temporal order of various disease manifestations. Of course, this view does not exclude the possibility that clinical heterogeneity represents "subtypes." For example, it is still conceivable that young onset disease or late onset disease, aphasic or other forms remain unique disease "subtypes." On the other hand, it is likely that these signs merely reflect a natural history of AD.

To further examine the progression to the final stages and death, we used a second Cox proportional hazards regression model with and without time-dependent covariates. This enabled us to use the survival analysis approach, but allowed us to enter "time-dependent" changes. In other words, we could evaluate and contrast the probability of surviving over time, given the presence of a single sign, such as psychosis, noted at the beginning of the disease and then evaluate the effect on the probability of dying by the emergence of other signs during follow-up. The Cox proportional hazard regression model with time-dependent covariates is a linear regression equivalent which is applied to censored data with binary outcomes, such as life or death. It allowed the examination of one clinical sign while controlling the other. It also allowed for the inclusion of covariates that vary with time, such as myoclonus or extrapyramidal signs. In this way we could examine three different models stratifying by the presence of extrapyramidal signs, myoclonus, or psychosis at the onset of the longitudinal study but could also utilize each sign as a time-dependent covariate considering the presence or development of these signs at any point during follow-up. Other potential predictors of mortality, such as age, duration of illness, functional or cognitive impairment, could be evaluated as a time-dependent measure. In the original cohort, 29 patients had died. Figure 1

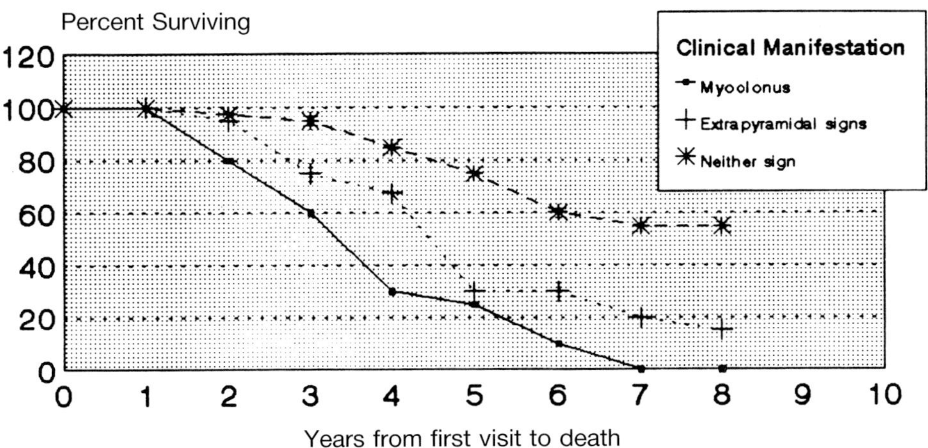

Fig. 1. Survival in patients with Alzheimer's disease. Comparison of those with myoclonus or extrapyramidal signs to those without either sign.[a]
[a] Does not correct for the presence of more than one sign.

illustrates the survival analyses for patients with either myoclonus or extrapyramidal signs at the onset. The differential survival rates noted for each were significantly different. In the Cox proportional hazards regression model, the risk of death in patients developing extrapyramidal signs was twice that for those who did not develop this sign. The risk of death in patients who develop myoclonus was 3.5 times that for those without these signs. However, when age, duration of illness, education, age of onset, and cognitive functional baseline values wee included in the model as fixed time covariates, only myoclonus had a unique value. In fact, when all signs were entered as time-dependent covariates, only myoclonus reached significance. The relative risk of dying for patients who develop myoclonus was three times that of patients who did not develop myoclonus. Extrapyramidal signs and psychosis did not reach significance in this analysis. In addition, and not unexpectedly, duration of disease, age, and functional decline at baseline were significant predictors of mortality. The survival analysis suggested that the presence of extrapyramidal signs or myoclonus early on predicts rapid progression of disease and early death. Using the Cox proportional hazard regression model we were able to determine whether the emergence of these signs during the patient's life would change the course of disease.

It has been suspected that the emergence of myoclonus might be related to disease duration. However, when entered as a time-dependent covariate, it is clear that myoclonus has predictive value over and above that related to disease progression. An alternate hypothesis is that the occurrence of myoclonus is predicted on a shorter span from that point to mortality. This hypothesis runs counter to the point raised by Drachman et al. (1990) which simply considers these clinical signs as related to disease duration rather than progression. However, the use of the Cox model would stroungly counter that view, particularly with regard to myoclonus.

Conclusions

Clinical heterogeneity probably plays an important role in the etiology and natural history of AD. Whether clinical heterogeneity represents phenotypic variation, pleiotropy or developmental stages of AD remains to be determined. Clearly, the information derived by the study of clinical heterogeneity in AD can be used to estimate stage of disease and prognosis. It may also be useful to identify particular phenotypes in order to establish specific etiologies.

Acknowledgments. This work was supported by Federal Grants AG07232, AG07370 and AG08702 and the Charles S. Robertson Memorial Gift for Alzheimer's Disease from the Banbury Fund.

References

Bird TD, Stranahan S, Sumi M, Raskind M (1983) Alzheimer's disease and choline acetyl-transferase activity in brain tissue form clinical and pathological subgroups. Ann Neurol 14:284–293

Breitner JCS, Folstein MF (1984) Familial Alzheimer dementia: a prevalent disorder with specific clinical features. Psychol Med 14:63–80

Breitner JCS, Murphy EA, Folstein MF (1986) Familial aggregation in Alzheimer Dementia-II. Clinical genetic implications of age-dependent onset. J Psych Res 20:45–55

Chartier-Harlin-M-C, Crawford F, Houlden H, Warren A, Hughes D, Fidani L, Goate A, Rossor M, Roques P, Hardy J, Mullan M, (1991) Early-onset Alzheimer's disease caused by mutations at codon 717 of the beta amyloid precursor protein gene. Nature 353:844–846

Chen J, Stern Y, Sano M, Mayeux R (1991) Cumulative risks of developing extrapyramidal signs, psychosis, and myoclonus in the course of Alzheimer's disease. Arch Neurol 48:1141–1146

Chui H, Teng EL, Henderson VW, Moy AC (1985) Clinical subtypes of dementia of the Alzheimer type. Neurology 35:1544–1550

Ditter SM, Mirra SS (1987) Neuropathologic and clinical features of Parkinson's disease in Alzheimer's disease patients. Neurology 37:754–760

Drachman DA, O'Donnell BF, Lew RA, Swearer JM (1990) The prognosis in Alzheimer's disease: "How far" rather than "how fast" best predicts the course. Arch Neurol 47:851–856

Duffy P, Mayeux R, Kupsky W (1988) Familial Alzheimer's disease with myoclonus and "spongy change". Arch Neurol 45:1097–1103

Goate A, Chartier-Harlin-M-C, Mullan M, Brown J, Crawford F, Fidani L, Giuffra L, Haynes A, Irving N, James L, Mant R, Newton P, Rooke K, Roques P, Talbot C, Pericak-Vance MA, Roses AD, Williamson R, Rossor M, Owen M, Hardy J (1991) Segregation of a missense mutation in the amyloid precursor protein gene with familial Alzheimer's disease. Nature 349:704–706

Heyman A, Wilkinson WE, Hurwitz BJ, Schmechel D, Sigmon AW, Weinberg T, Helms MJ, Swist M (1983) Alzheimer's disease: genetic aspects and associated clinical disorders. Ann Neurol 14:507–515

Jorm AF (1985) Subtypes of Alzheimer's dementia: a conceptual analysis and critical review. Psych Med 15:543–553

Kaye JA, May C, Atack JR, Daly E, Sweeny DL, Beal MF, Kaufman S, Milstien S, Friedland RP, Rapoport SI (1988a) Cerebrospinal fluid neurochemistry in the myoclonic subtype of Alzheimer's disease. Ann Neurol 24:647–650

Kaye JA, May C, Daly E, Atack JR, Sweeny DL, Luxenberg JS, Kay AD, Kaufman S, Milstien S, Friedland RP, Rapoport SI (1988b) Cerebrospinal fluid monoamine markers are decreased in dementia of the Alzheimer type with extrapyramidal features. Neurology 38:554–557

Lucotte G, Berriche S, David F (1991) Alzheimer's mutations. Nature 351:530

Mayeux R, Stern Y, Spanton S (1985) Heterogeneity in dementias of the Alzheimer type: Evidence for subgroups. Neurology 35:453–461

Murrell J, Farlow M, Ghetti B, Benson MD (1991) A mutation in the amyloid precursor protein associated with hereditary Alzheimer's disease. Science 254:97–99

Naruse S, Igarashi S, Kobayashi H, Aoki K, Inuzuka T, Kaneko K, Shimizu T, Jihara K, Kojima T, Miyatake T, Tsuji S (1991) Mis-sense mutation Val → Ile in exon 17 of amyloid precursor protein gene in Japanese familial Alzheimer's disease. Lancet 337:1342–1343

Pericak-Vance MA, Bebout JL, Gaskell PC Jr, Yamaoka LH, Hung W-Y, Alberts MJ, Walker AP, Bartlett RJ, Haynes CA, Welsh KA, Earl NL, Heyman A, Clark Cam, Roses AD (1991) Linkage studies in familial Alzheimer's disease, application of affected pedigree member method of linkage analysis. Am J Human Genet 48:1034–1050

Seltzer B, Sherwin I (1983) A comparison of clinical features in early- and late-onset primary degenerative dementia. Arch Neurol 40:143–146

Stern Y, Hesdorffer D, Sano M, Mayeux R (1990) Measurement and prediction of functional capacity in Alzheimer's disease. Neurology 40:8–13

Stern Y, Mayeux R, Sano M, Hauser WA, Bush T (1987) Predictors of disease course in patients with probable Alzheimer's disease. Neurology 37:1649–1653

St George-Hyslop PH, Tanzi RE, Polinsky RJ, Haines JL, Nee L, Watkins PC, Myers RH, Feldman RG, Pollen D, Drachmann D, Growdon J, Bruni A, Foncin J-F, Salmon D, Frommelt P, Amaducci L, Sorbi S, Piacentini S, Stewart GD, Hobbs WJ, Conneally PM, Gusella JF (1987) The genetic defect causing familial Alzheimer's disease maps on chromosome 21. Science 235:885–890

St George-Hyslop PH, Haines JL, Farrer LA, Polinsky R, Van Broeckhoven C, Goate A, Crapper McLachlan DR, Orr H, Bruni AC, Sorbi S, Rainero I, Foncin JF, Pollen D, Cantu J-M, Tupler R, Voskresenskaya N, Mayeux R, Growdon J, Fried VA, Myers RH, Nee L, Backhovens H, Martin J-J, Rossor M, Owen MJ, Mullan M, Percy ME, Karlinsky K, Rich S, Heston L, Montesi M, Mortilla M, Nacmias N, Gusella JF (1990) Genetic linkage studies suggest Alzheimer's disease is not a single homogeneous disorder. Nature 347:194–196

Prognostic Implications of Symptomatic Behaviors in Alzheimer's Disease

H. C. Chui, S. Lyness, E. Sobel, and *L. S. Schneider*

Summary

Symptomatic behaviors frequently accompany Alzheimer's disease (AD) and include disturbances of mood, perception, and motor activity. The frequency of such symptoms reported in the literature varies depending upon symptom definition and stage of illness, but usually ranges between 20 to 40%. The biological bases that underlie these disturbances are not well understood, but probably related to the presence of specific pathological and neurochemical substrates (e.g., disproportionate pathology in limbic/paralimbic structures of the frontal-temporal lobes or changes in biogenic amine systems). A number of investigators, using different strategies and analytic methods, have shown that symptomatic behaviors are associated with a faster rate of cognitive decline. The biological significance of this association between behavior and cognition is unknown. It is conceivable, however, that the same distribution of pathologic lesions and neurochemical changes that predispose to psychosis may also hasten the rate of cognitive decline.

Introduction

Symptomatic behaviors are frequently associated with dementing disorders such as Alzheimer's disease (AD). These symptoms include changes in personality, mood, perception, thinking, and motor activity (Larson et al., 1963; Gustafson, 1975; Reisberg et al., 1987). These disturbances may be more disruptive to daily function and more troublesome to caregiving than cognitive loss, per se (Rabins et al., 1982); they are often important risk factors for institutionalization (Steele et al., 1990).

In this paper, we review the epidemiology, biology and prognostic implications of psychosis and agitation, two symptomatic behaviors characteristic of AD. Changes in personality and disturbances of mood (e.g., anxiety and depression) are not included. Also, even though behavioral symptoms may at times be amenable to treatment, interventional issues fall outside the scope of this paper.

F. Boller et al. (Eds.)
Heterogeneity of Alzheimer's Disease
© Springer-Verlag Berlin Heidelberg 1992

Definitions

The key component of psychosis is a disturbance in reality testing. Psychotic symptoms include disorders of perception (hallucinations) and thinking (delusions); they may also include disorders of identification. Hallucinations refer to "sensory without external stimulation of the relevant sensory organ" (DSM-IIIR 1987). Visual and auditory hallucinations are commonly reported in patients with AD (for review, see Wragg and Jeste, 1989; Burns, 1990b).

Delusions are "false personal belief(s) based on incorrect inference about external reality and firmly sustained in spite of what almost everyone else believes and in spite of what constitutes incontrovertible and obvious proof or evidence to the contrary" (DSM-IIIR 1987). In AD, delusions tend to be simple, loosely structured beliefs, often with persecutory content (e.g., belief that possessions have been stolen, or that one's spouse is unfaithful; Cummings, 1985; for review see Wragg and Jeste, 1989). Delusional material also can be interpreted as a product of memory loss (Reisberg et al., 1987). For example, the belief that objects have been stolen may result from failing to remember where they had been placed.

Misidentifications refer to the mistaken recognition or belief about what is perceived. Patients with AD may insist that their spouse is an imposter (Capgras syndrome), fail to recognize their own image in the mirror, or mistake TV images for real people. Misidentifications may result from a combination of disturbances in perception, memory cognition and reality testing. Persistent misidentifications are usually associated with paranoid delusions (Rosen and Zubenko, 1991).

Agitation is used broadly to refer to several types of increased motor activity with normal form (Victoroff, 1989). It may range from hyperactivity (e.g., restlessness, pacing, wandering, non-specific agitation; Victoroff, 1989) to either verbally of physically aggressive acts directed at objects or other persons (Swearer et al., 1988; Deutsch et al., 1991).

Frequency of Symptomatic Behaviors in AD

The frequences of hallucinations, delusions, misidentifications and agitation occuring in AD patients and reported in the post-1985 literature are summarized in Table 1. The crude prevalences are relatively consistent (e.g., for hallucinations and delusions, between 16 and 33% in 11 of 12 studies). Methologic issues, however, such as patient sampling, method of ascertainment, stage of illness, and period of survey time contribute to the variability in the relative frequencies. Agitation has been more commonly reported among patients living in the nursing home (Cohen-Mansfield, 1986) than in the community (Rubin et al., 1987). Inclusion of misidentifications as a delusional symptom increases the frequency of psychosis. Higher symptom frequencies are found when data are derived from caregivers rather than patient responses. Symptomatic behaviors are more common in certain stages of dementia. Finally, the cumulative frequency of symptoms increases with the duration of the survey

Table 1. Relative Frequency (%) of symptomatic behaviors in Alzheimer's disease reported in the literature since 1985

	n	Delu-sions	Halluci-nations	Misiden-tifica-tions	Agita-tion	Dura-tion	Severity of dementia[a]
Cohen-Mansfield, 1986	66[b]	–	–	–	73	–	BCRS =5.9
Robin et al. 1987[c]	44	–	–	25–67	32	–	CDR = 0.5–1.0
Cummings et al. 1987	30	47	3[d]	–	–	–	MMSE = 1.46 (1.9)
Reisberg et al. 1987	57	12	24	48	–	–	GDS ≥ 4
Rubin et al. 1988	110	31	25	23	–	–	–
Teri et al. 1988	127	24	21	–	24	–	MMSE = 17
Merriam et al. 1988	175	24	28	49	61	4.5	BIMCT = 18.6
Teri et al. 1990[c]	106	22	25	–	21	3.9	MMSE = 18.2 (6.7)
Burns et al. 1990	178	16	23	23	–	5.2	–
Mendez et al. 1990	217	30	25	17	–	3.3	MMSE = 17.2 (6.5)
+ Cooper et al. 1990	677	26	17	–	–	–	MMSE = 13.6 (8.3)
Rosen & Zubenko 1991[c]	32[e]	34	31	–	–	5.3	MMSE = 13.7
Deutsch et al. 1991	181	44	24	30	–	–	MMSE =11.9 (6.7)
Jeste et al. 1992[c]	107	35	17	–	–	4.3	–
mean		29	22	31	42		
s.d.		10.3	7.2	12.7	23.4		
number of studies		12	12	7	5		
number of patients		2027	2027	962	518		

[a] Abbreviations: BCRS, Brief Cognitive Rating Scale; CDR, Clinical Dementia Rating; MMSE, Mini-Mental State Examinations, BIMCT, Blessed Information Memory Concentration Test
[b] Nursing home
[c] Iongitudinal study
[d] direct patient interview
[e] Autopsy confirmed

period (Drevets and Rubins, 1989; Rosen and Zubenko, 1991; Chen et al., 1991).

Inter-correlations between various types of symptomatic behaviors may indicate the likelihood of common underlying pathogenetic mechanisms. Delusions and hallucinations frequently coexist in the same patients (Cooper et al., 1991; for review, see Wragg and Jeste, 1989) and can occur independently (Burns et al., 1990; Rosen and Zubenko, 1991). Some associations have been reported between psychosis and agitation (Cooper et al., 1991) or aggression (Lopez et al., 1991; Deutsch et al., 1991). In our own studies, significant correlations have been found between delusions and hallucinations, but neither psychotic symptom correlated with agitation (Chui et al., submitted). Taken together, these data suggest that similar pathogenetic mechanisms may give rise to delusions and hallucinations, whereas a distinct pathologic substrate may lead to agitation.

Given the high frequency of symptomatic behaviors in AD, it is reasonable to question whether they represent a distinct subgroup of disease or a manifestation of a certain stage of illness. To some extent, the development of these symptoms is stage-related, with cumulative rates increasing throughout the mild, moderate and severe stages of dementia (Chen et al., 1991; Rosen and Zubenko, 1991). In far advanced stages, however, psychotic symptoms often resolve. Possible reasons include progressive loss of the brain substrate necessary to sustain these symptoms, the inability of patients to express ongoing symptoms, or the inability to clinically detect these symptoms (Cummings et al., 1987; Rosen and Zubenko, 1991).

Despite the increasing rate of symptoms, the relationship between symptomatic behaviors and duration or severity of illness is not a strong one. In one study, duration of illness was not significantly related to the development of hallucinations or misidentifications (Burns et al., 1990). Inconsistent relationships have been reported between symptom frequency and severity of dementia. For psychosis, no significant associations (Teri et al., 1988), a negative trend (Cummings et al., 1987), positive correlations (Swearer et al., 1988; Cooper et al., 1991; Rosen and Zubenko, 1991), or mixed associations (Merriam et al., 1988; Burns et al., 1990a, b) have been reported. For motor symptoms, wandering and agitation, but not restlessness have been correlated with cognitive decline (Teri et al., 1988). Only weak correlations between troublesome and disruptive behaviors and severity of dementia have been noted in another report (Swearer et al., 1988). Finally, in two longitudinal studies approximately half of the AD patients developed psychotic symptoms sometime during their disease course while half did not (Chen et al., 1991; Rosen and Zubenko, 1991). Thus, while the appearance of symptomatic behaviors is partially related to stage of illness, other biological factors probably contribute to the likelihood of their occurrence.

Biological basis for Symptomatic Behaviors

Little is known about the anatomical and biochemical bases for symptomatic behaviors in AD. Several neurobehavioral models, however, have been proposed to explain the pathogenesis of delusions (Cummings, 1985) and hyperactivity (Victoroff, 1989). Lesions of the limbic system or its interconnections have been postulated to give rise to abnormal emotional experiences (Cummings et al., 1987). Interactions between these altered experiences and available intellect might lead to delusional thinking. When the cerebral hemispheres are intact, complex delusions may be elaborated. On the other hand, when the cerebral hemispheres are damaged, as in AD, simple delusions result.

An anatomical circuit by which the limbic system may modulate the level of motor activity has also been proposed (Victoroff, 1989). The major structures involved in this circuit include the hippocampus, nucleus accumbens, basal forebrain, and the mesencephalic locomotor region. Two of these structures, namely the hippocampus and basal forebrain, are highly vulnerable to developing AD pathology. Litte has been written about the anatomical basis for hallucinations or misidentifications, although one might speculate about the role of pathologic lesions in sensory association areas.

To date, no characteristic anatomical pattern of atrophy has been noted in neuroimaging studies of patients with symptomatic behaviors. Using univariate analyses, Jacoby an and Levy, 1980) reported an inverse correlation between paranoid delusions and a cortical atrophy index score, but this finding could not be confirmed in subsequent studies (Burns et al., 1990a). Quantitative-correlative studies of limbic, paralimbic and frontal-temporal association areas have yet to be done.

Jeste et al. (1992) found that, despite equivalent age, education and duration of illness, AD patients with delusions were significantly more impaired on neuropsychological testing, particularly in the areas of conceptualization and memory. For a subset of mildly demented patients, those with delusions tended to be more impaired on the Wisconsin Card Sort and the similarities subtest of the Wechsler Adult Intelligence Scale, two tests purportedly sensitive to prefrontal lobe deficits. These investigators have suggested that the development of delusional symptoms results from pathology in the frontal-temporal regions of the brain. Recently, abnormalities in these brain regions have been reported in patients with functional psychoses such as schizophrenia (Suddath et al., 1989).

Neuropathologic studies have also suggested that certain areas within the temporal and frontal lobes may be differentialy involved in AD. Zubenko et al. (1991) found that patients with psychosis had significantly more senile plaques in prosubiculum and neurofibrillary tangles in mid-frontal cortex than patients without psychosis, although there was considerable overlap. These authors also reported that psychotic patients had lower levels of 5-hydroxytryptamine in the prosubiculum, whereas non-psychotic patients had lower concentrations of norepinephrine in the substantia nigra. Thus, not only anatomical, but also specific biochemical abnormalities may predispose to the development of psychosis.

The binding site for ^{3}H-imipramine is associated with serotonin uptake; its localization in the brain parallels the distribution of serotonergic innervation (Langer et al., 1981). Decreases in brain ^{3}H-imipramine binding density have been demonstrated in post-mortem AD specimens from caudate, hypothalamus (Carlsson et al., 1980) and temporal lobes (Bowen et al., 1983). Since platelet ^{3}H-imipramine binding shares many characteristics of the brain binding site, it has been examined as a potential peripheral marker for various neuropsychiatric disorders (Mellerup and Langer, 1990).

We have reported significantly lower B_{max} values for platelet ^{3}H-imipramine binding density in a subset of AD patients with symptomatic behaviors (agitation or delusions) compared either to AD subjects without these behaviors or to normal controls (Schneider et al., 1988). Other investigators have not found any differences in platelet ^{3}H-imipramine binding in AD patients compared to normal controls (Suranyi-Cadotte et al., 1985; Galzin et al., 1989), however, AD patients with delusions were not selected for comparison. The finding of differences in platelet ^{3}H-imipramine binding in a subset of AD patients warrants replication; it could suggest a contributory role for serotonergic or other biogenic amines systems in the genesis of symptomatic behaviors.

Table 2. Symptomatic behaviors and rate of progression in AD.comparison of dementia severity at follow-up

First Author	Sample (n)	Follow-up Interval (total F/U in yr)	Method	Independent variable (non-sign predictor)	Dependent variable[a]
Drevets 1989	67	Fixed (5.5)	Student's t	psychosis	CDR DS, DSC, SPMSQ
Burns 1990	178	Fixed (1.0)	Student's t	hallucinations (delusions) (misidentifications)	MMSE CAMCOG
Teri 1990	106	Variable (0.92)	2-stage random effect regression	agitation alcohol neurological disease (9 other behavior and 4 other health problems	MMSE
Lopez 1991	34	Fixed (1.0)	ANOVA	psychosis	MMSE Neuropsychiatric test
Rosen 1991	32	Variable (0 ko 5)	Student's t	psychosis	MMSE

[a] Abbreviations: MMSE, Mini-Mental State Examination; CDR, Clinical Dementia Rating; DS, Blessed Dementia Scale; DSC, Blessed Dementia Scale-Cognitive; SPMSQ, Short Portable Mental Status Questionnaire; CAMCOG, CAMDEX cognitive assessment

Association between Symptomatic Behaviors and Rate of dementia Progression

Several investigators have examined the association between symptomatic behaviors and the rate of dementia progression in AD. Although there are exceptions (Teri et al., 1990), in general, two study designs have been employed:
1. patients are matched for severity of dementia at study entry and are followed at regular intervals; t-tests or ANOVA are used to compare dementia severity at each fixed follow-up interval (Table 2);
2. patients who present with varying severity of dementia at initial evaluation and who are followed at various time intervals are assessed using survival analyses (Table 3).

The Kaplan-Meier model compares survival curves for univariate categorical predictors (e.g., psychotic vs non-psychotic), while the Cox proportional hazards model allows comparison of the relative prognostic power of multivariate factors (e.g., age at onset, psychosis, extrapyramidal, etc.).

Comparison of dementia severity at follow-up

Drevets and Rubins (1989) followed mildly demented subjects with early psychotic symptoms (n = 10) versus without early psychosis (n = 15) at regular

Table 3. Symptomatic behaviors and rate of progression in AD. survival analyses[a]

First Author	Sample (n)	Follow-up Interval (total F/U in yr)	Method	Significant Predictor (non-sign predictor)	Endpoint
Stern1987	65	Variable (2.8 ± 1.6)	Kaplan Meier	psychosis[b] EPS[b]	mMMSE score < 20 BDRS > 15
Drachman 1990	42	Variable (4.5 ± 2.1)	Kaplan-Meier Cox	7 severity factors (10 other factors, including psychosis, age, education, family history)	total dependence ADL incontinence institutionalization
Chui 1992	113	Variable (2.5 ± 1.8)	Cox		
	total sample (n = 113)			Initial MMSE (8 other factors)	MMSE = 10
	mild dementia (n = 61)			hallucinations[c]	
	moderate dementia (n = 52)			extrapyramidal	
	total sample			agitation[c] extrapyramidal[c]	5-point drop in MMSE
	mild dementia			agitation hallucinations	
	moderate dementia			delusions	

[a] Abbreviations: MMSE, Mini-Mental State Examination; mMMSE, modified Mini-Mental State Examination; BDRS, Blessed Dementia Rating Scale; EPS, extrapyramidal signs; ADL, activities of daily living

[b] trend suggesting shorter survival to cognitive (mMMSE), but not functional, (BDRS) endpoint

[c] $p < 0.07$

intervals over 66 months. By 15 months, the psychotic group had deteriorated more rapidly in cognitive function, functional ability, and clinical dementia rating than the non-psychotic group.

In a study of 178 patients with probable or possible AD drawn an epidemiologic catchment area, Burns et al. (1990a) reported that the presence of hallucinations at initial visit was associated with greater deterioration in cognitive function over the ensuing 12 months. Delusions and misidentifications, on the other hand, did not predict a faster rate of decline.

Teri et al. (1990) studies 106 patients with primary degenerative dementia who were given the Mini-Mental State Examination (MMSE) one to five times over up to three years. A two-stage random effects' regression model was fit to the data and then used to assess the effects of behavioral, health and descriptive measures on the rate of decline. Agitation as well as alcohol abuse and the presence of additional neurological disease were associated with significantly faster rates of cognitive decline.

In another study, 17 AD patients with delusions and hallucinations were matched for education, initial MMSE, severity and duration of illness with 17 without these symptoms and were followed for one year (Lopez et al., 1991). At the time of entry into the study, the AD patients with psychosis showed a specific defect in receptive language, had a higher frequency of associated aggression and hostility, and electroencephalographic abnormalities. The patients with psychotic symptoms showed a significantly more rapid rate of decline in MMSE.

Rosen and Zubenko (1991) studied 32 dementia patients with definite, histopathologically confirmed AD. Over a follow-up period of zero to five years, psychosis emerged in 15 (47%) and major depressive episode in seven patients (22%). The occurrence of psychosis at any time during the natural history was associated with more rapid cognitive decline on the MMSE (one-tailed t test), but not with increased mortality. The mean initial MMSE was also lower for the psychotic group (13.7 ± 8.3) than for the non-psychotic group (17.0 ± 8.5), but this was apparently not significant.

In summary, five independent studies since 1989 have reported significantly greater severity of dementia at follow-up for those patients with symptomatic behaviors at the time of initial evaluation. The focus in four of these studies was upon psychotic symptoms; in one study using multivariate regression analyses, agitation rather than psychosis was the significant predictor (Teri et al., 1990).

Survival analyses

Two survival analyses with different results have been reported in the literature (Stern et al., 1987; Drachmann et al., 1990), a third study (Chui et al., submitted) is also described here (Table 3). Stern et al. (1987) followed 65 patients with probable AD at various intervals for up to 7.1 years (mean 2.8 ± 1.6). All patients were seen at least twice, with a minimum follow-up interval of six months. The Kaplan-Meier product limit technique was used to describe the probability that patients in certain subgroups would reach an endpoint as a function of duration of illness. The presence or absence of psychiatric symptoms (persistent hallucinations, illusions, or delusions) or extrapyramidal signs at the initial clinic visit was used to define patient subgroups. Scores on a cognitive (modified MMSE) and a functional (Blessed Activities of Daily Living) rating scale served as endpoint. A trend was found showing that either psychosis or extrapyramidal disorder was associated with a higher probability of reaching the cognitive, but not functional, endpoint.

In a "negative" study (Drachman et al., 1990), 42 patients with probable AD were followed longitudinally over a mean period of 4.5 years (s.d. = 2.1). Both Kaplan-Meier and Cox proportional hazards (p < 0.01) analyses were used to assess the power of several variables to predict survival to three fixed functional endpoints (total dependence in activites of daily living, incontinence, or institutionalization). During the follow-up period, from 74 to 80% of the patients had reached each one of the endpoints. Measures of initial dementia severity (e.g., clinical dementia rating, performance on subtests of the WAIS-R or WMS) were significant predictors of decreased survival to endpoint. The presence of extrapyramidal signs or psychotic symptoms at initial visit was not. These investigators concluded that "how far" rather than "how fast" best predicts the clinical course of AD.

Our own data (Chui et al., submitted) corroborate the association between symptomatic behaviors and faster rate of dementia progression. Rate of progression was analysed using a Cox proportional hazards models in 113 patients who met all three of the following inclusion criteria:

1. diagnosis of either definite (n = 9) or probably AD (n = 104; McKhann et al., 1984);
2. initial MMSE $\geq$ 15; and
3. at least one follow-up MMSE performed at least one month after the initial evaluation.

The total sample was divided into two subgroups with either mild (MMSE from 20 to 28) or moderate (MMSE from 15 to 19) dementia. Nine predictor variables included: initial MMSE scores, gender, education, age at symptom onset, family history of dementia, presence of hallucinations, delusions, agitation, and presence of extrapyramidal signs while not on neuroleptics. Two cognitive endpoints were defined:

1. arrival at a fixed MMSE score of 10 and
2. decline in MMSE score of 5 points.

Forty percent of the 113 patients reached the fixed endpoint of MMSE = 10 over a median follow-up period of 75 weeks (range = 8–293 weeks). In this model, the only significant predictor of reaching endpoint was the initial MMSE (i.e., patients with higher initial MMSE had a smaller likelihood of reaching endpoint). These findings replicate those of Drachman et al., 1990), who reported that "how far" rather than "how fast" was the best predictor of outcome. When the sample was divided into mild and moderate dementia subgroups, however, hallucinations (risk-hazard ratio = 4.1) and extrapyramidal signs (risk-hazard ratio = 11.2) were associated with a faster rate of progression. Reduced variability in initial MMSE within the two subgroups may have permitted the detection of significant risk factors.

When an individual's endpoint was taken as a 5-point decline in MMSE score from baseline, inter-individual differences in initial severity of dementia were effectively normalized. Sixty-eight percent of the 113 patients reached this endpoint over a median follow-up period of 48 weeks (ranging from 6 to 254 weeks). Within two subgroups of patients with mild and moderate dementia, several variables proved to be statistically significant (p < 0.05) predictors of decreased "survival," i.e., faster rate of progression. In the mildly demented group, these variables were agitation and hallucinations (risk/hazard ratios were 4.6 and 5.1, respectively). In the moderately demented group, delusions at initial entry predicted decreased survival (risk/hazard ratio, 3.4. Within the entire dementia group, multivariate results showed a statistical trend (p < 0.10) suggesting that several non-cognitive symptoms such as extrapyramidal signs and agitation were significant predictors of deterioration.

In conclusion, when initial severity of MMSE is "controlled," either by dividing the sample into subgroups or by defining the endpoint as a 5-point decline in MMSE, several symptomatic behaviors (delusions, hallucinations, agitation) as well as extrapyramidal signs predict a faster rate of cognitive decline. At the present time, the independence of these predictors can be questioned; significant correlations were found between hallucinations and delusions, and delusions and extrapyramidal signs, although not between agitation and the other factors. The biological explanation for these associations between behavior and cognition is not known. While it is possible that the presence of psychosis increases confusion, patients are usually not floridly psychotic during testing (Jeste et al., 1992). Since the majority of patients with symptomatic behaviors are treated empirically with psychotropic medications, drug side-effects may adversely affect cognition (Devanand et al., 1989). Finally, the very distribution of pathologic lesions and neurochemical changes that may predispose to psychosis may also hasten the rate of cognitive decline.

Acknowledgment. This work is supported by the National Institutes of Aging (1P50 AG05142) and the State of California Department of Health Services (Alzheimer Disease Diagnostic and Treatment Centers).

References

American Psychiatric Association (1987) Diagnostic and Statistical Manual of Mental Disorders-Revised 3rd ed. Washington, D. C.: American Psychiatric Association.

Bowen DM, Allen SJ, Benton JS, Goodhardt MJ, Haan EA, Palmer AM, Sins NR, Smith CC, Spillane JA, Esiri MM, Neary D, Snowdon JS, Wilcock GK, Davison AN (1983) Biochemical assessment of serotonergic and cholinergic dysfunction and cerebral atrophy in Alzheimer's disease. J Neurochem 41:266–272

Burns A, Jacoby R, Levy R (1990a) Psychiatric phenomena in Alzheimer's disease. I: disorders of thought content. Brit J Psychiat 157:72–76

Burns A, Jacoby R, Levy (1990b) Psychiatric phenomena in Alzheimer's disease. II. Disorders of perception. Brit J Psychiat 157:76–81

Carlsson A, Adofsson R, Aquilonius S-M, Goffries CG, Oreland L, Svennerholm L, Winblad B (1980) Biogenic amines in human brain in normal aging, senile dementia and chronic alcoholism. In: Goldstein M et al. (eds) Ergot compounds and brain function: neuroendocrine and neuropsychiatric aspects. New York, Raven Press, pp 295–304

Chen JY, Stern Y, Sano M, Mayeux R (1991) Cumulative risks of developing extrapyramidal signs, psychosis, or myoclonus in the course of Alzheimer's disease. Arch Neurol 48:1141–1143

Cohen-Mansfield J (1986) Agitated behaviors in the elderly. II. Preliminary results in the cognitively deteriorated. J Am Geriatr Soc 34:722–727

Cooper JK, Mungas D, Verma M, Weiler P (1991) Psychotic symptoms in Alzheimer's disease. Internat J Ger Psychiat 6:721–726

Cummings JL (1985) Organic delusions: Phenomenology, anatomical correlations, and review. Brit J Psychiat 146:184–197

Cummings JL, Miller B, Hill MA, Neshkes R (1987) Neuropsychiatric aspects of multi-infarct dementia and dementia of Alzheimer type. Arch Neurol 37:1649–1653

Deutsch LH, Bylsma FW, Rovner BW, Steele C, Folstein MF (1991) Psychosis and physical aggression in probable Alzheimer's disease. Am J Psychiat 148:1159–1163

Devanand DP, Sackheim HA, Brown RP, Mayeux R (1989) A pilot study of haloperidol treatment of psychosis and behavioral disturbance in Alzheimer disease. Arch Neurol 46:854–857

Drachman DA, O'Donnell BF, Lew RA, Swearer JM (1990) The prognosis in Alzheimer's disease: "How far" rather than "how fast" best predicts the course. Arch Neurol 47:851–856

Drevets WC, Rubins EH (1989) Psychotic symptoms and the longitudinal course of senile dementia of Alzheimer type. Biol Psychiat 25:39–48

Galzin AM, Davous P, Roudier M, Lamour Y, Poirier M-F, Langer S (1989) Platelet [^{3}H-]- · imipramine binding is not modified in Alzheimer's disease. Psychiat Res 28:289–294

Gustafson L (1975) Psychiatric symptoms in dementia with onset in the presenile period. Acta Psychiat Scand 257 (suppl):8–35

Jacoby RJ, Levy R (1980) Computed tomography in the elderly. 2. Senile dementia: diagnosis and functional impairment. Brit J Psychiat 136:256–269

Jeste DV, Wragg RE, Salmon DP, Harris MJ, Tahl LJ (1992) Cognitive deficits of patients with Alzheimer's disease with and without delusions. Am J Psychiat 149:184–189

Langer SZ, Javoy-Agid F, Raisman R, Briley MS, Agid Y (1981) Distribution of specific high-affinity binding sites for ^{3}H-imipramine in human brain. J Neurochem 37:267–271

Larson T, Sjogren T, Jacobson G (1963) Senile dementia. Acta Psychiat Scand 167 (Suppl):1–259

Lopez OL, Becker JT, Brenner RP, Rosen J, Bajulaiye Ol, Reynolds CF (1991) Alzheimer's disease with delusions and hallucinations: neuropsychological and electroencephalographic correlates. Neurology 41:906–912

McKhann G, Drachman D, Folstein M, Katzman R, Price D, Stadlan EM (1984) Clinical diagnosis of Alzheimer's disease: report of the NINCDS-ADRDA Work Group under the auspices of Department of Health and Human Services Task Force on Alzheimer's disease. Neurology 34:939–944

Mellerup E, Langer SZ (1990) Validity of impipramine platelet binding sites as a biological marker of endogenous depression: a World Health Organization collaborative study. Pharmacopsychiatry 23:113–117

Mendez MF, Martin RJ, Smyth KA, Whitehouse PJ (1990) Psychiatric symptoms associated with Alzheimer's disease. Neuropsychiat Clin Neurosci 2:28–33

Merriam AE, Aronson MK, Gaston P, Wey S, Katz I (1988) The psychiatric symptoms of Alzheimer's disease. J Am Ger Soc 36:7–12

Rabins PV, Mace NL, Lucas MJ (1982) The impact of dementia on the family. JAMA 248:333–335

Reisberg B, Borenstein J, Salob S, Ferris SH, Franssen E, Gorgotas A (1987) Behavioral symptoms in Alzheimer's disease: phenomenology and treatment. J Clin Psych 48 (5, suppl):9–15

Rosen J, Zubenko GS (1991) Emergence of psychosis and depression in the longitudinal evaluation of Alzheimer's disease. Biol Psychiat 29:224–232

Rubin EH, Morris JC, Storandt M, Berg L (1987) Behavioral changes in patients with mild senile dementia of the Alzheimer's type. Psychiat Res 21:55–62

Rubin EH, Drevets WC, Burke WJ (1988) The nature of psychotic symptoms in senile dementia of the Alzheimer type. J Geriatr Psych Neurol 1:16–20

Schneider LS, Severson JA, Chui HC, Pollock VE, Sloane RB, Fredrickson ER (1988) Platelet tritiated imipramine binding and MAO activity in Alzheimer's disease patients with agitation and delusions. Psychiat Res 25:311–322

Steele C, Rovner B, Chase GA, Folstein M (1990) Psychiatric symptoms and nursing home placement of patients with Alzheimer's disease. Am J Psychiat 147:1049–1051

Stern Y, Mayeux R, Sano M, Hause WA, Bush T (1987) Predictors of disease course in patients with probable Alzheimer's disease. Neurology 37:1649–1653

Suddath RL, Casanova MF, Goldberg RE, Daniel DG, Kelsoe JR Jr, Weinberger DR (1989) Temporal lobe pathology in schizophrenia: a quantitative magnetic resonance imaging study. Am J Psychat 146:464–472

Suranyi-Cadotte BE, Gauthier S, Lafaille F, DeFlores S., Dam TV, Naip NP, Quirion R (1985) Platelet ^{3}H-imipramine binding distinguishes depression from Alzheimer dementia. Life Sci 37:2305–2311

Swearer JM, Drachman DA, O'Donnell BF, Mitchell AL (1988) Troublesome and disruptive behaviors in dementia. J Am Geriatr Soc 36:784–790

Teri L, Larson EB, Reifler BV (1988) Behavioral disturbance in dementia of the Alzheimer's type. J Am Ger Soc 36:1–6

Teri L, Hughes JP, Larson EB (1990) Cognitive deterioration in Alzheimer's disease: Behavioral and health factors. J Geron 45:58–63

Victoroff JI (1989) Hyperactivity syndrome in Alzheimer's disease. Bull Clin Neurosci 53:-34–42

Wragg RE, Jeste DV (1989) Overview of depression and psychosis in Alzheimer's disease. Am J Psychiat 146:1182–1186

Zubenko GS, Moossy J, Martinez AJ, Rao G, Claassen D, Rosen J, Kopp U (1991) Neuropathologic and Neurochemical Correlates of Psychosis in Primary Dementia. Arch Neurol 48:619–624

Heterogeneous Disappearance of Knowledge in Alzheimer's Disease

J. Grafman

Summary

The heterogeneity of Alzheimer's disease (AD) can be utilized by neurobehavioral researchers interested in making a contribution to our understanding of the functional architecture concerned with knowledge representation. I will illustrate two aspects of knowledge disappearance in AD by describing two patients: one with a progressive loss of number processing and calculation ability and a second patient with a relatively selective loss of body schema knowledge. These two cases, in conjunction with a larger body of knowledge regarding the ability of AD patients to retrieve various types, and aspects, of learned knowledge, argue for the functional heterogeneity of AD.

Introduction

The progressive cognitive deficits that are the hallmark of Alzheimer's disease (AD) are tragic. Not only does the patient become less able to remember day-to-day events, but eventually even old learned knowledge becomes inaccessible for conscious deliberation, understanding, and expression. At this stage of the disease, patients may not recognize their spouse of forty years or their children. It was once thought that the progression of neuropsychological deficits in AD was relatively orderly, with mild memory deficits leading to more severe ones, followed by a cascading loss of word finding, gnosic, and praxis skills, with language recognition and gestural communication the last cognitive abilities to be affected (McKhann et al., 1984). In turn, the pathologic process in AD was also seen to be orderly and focused in the hippocampus and posterior association cortex (Van Hoesen and Damasio, 1987).

However, over the last ten years, a more complicated picture of the AD patient has emerged that shows frequent neuropsychologic and pathologic deviation from the classical progression. In these studies, selective deficits can be found (Martin, 1987; Martin et al., 1986; Schwartz, 1990). Moreover, these deficits are persistent and, in some cases, may remain selective until the death of the patient (Schwartz and Chawluk, 1990). For example, Martin et al. (1986) found at least three separate subgroups of AD patients in their study. One group was generally impaired, another group had predominantly verbal deficits, and the last group demonstrated primarily visual-construction deficits.

F. Boller et al. (Eds.)
Heterogeneity of Alzheimer's Disease
© Springer-Verlag Berlin Heidelberg 1992

Interestingly, on follow-up, Martin et al. found that the profile of deterioration was group-dependent. That is, the verbal deficit group continued to decline predominantly in the verbal sphere, the visual-construction deficit group in the visual sphere, and the generalized deficit group declined across-the-board.

Haxby (1990) studied AD patients using positron emission tomography (PET) scans. PET studies have routinely identified asymmetric hypometabolic flow patterns. Haxby was able to show that the left-right and anterior-posterior distributions in such asymmetric patterns were correlated with performance on specific neuropsychological tests. For example, he found that performance on a test of attention correlated most with anterior hypometabolism, and performance on verbal tests correlated most with left hemisphere hypometabolism. These findings, while expected, strongly argue that the neuropsychological profile in AD is a direct result of distinct regional patterns of pathology (Celsis et al., 1987).

Neuropathological investigations have sometimes revealed that a subgroup of suspected AD patients with such selective cognitive deficits had focal, but non-AD, pathology (Kobayashi et al., 1990). However, other subgroups of patients with neuropathologically confirmed AD also demonstrated selective deficits that either persisted to the late stages of the disease or, for a limited period, revealed dissociations in cognitive performance that heretofore were unsuspected to exist so clearly in patients with AD (Poeck and Luzzatti, 1988; Pogacar and Williams, 1984). For example, Morrison and colleagues (Hof et al., 1989; Morrison et al., 1991) have examined neuropathological data in AD patients who presented with Balint's syndrome. The analysis yielded a strong correlation between the distribution of plaques and neurofibrillary tangles in specific visual pathways and the presence of the visual deficits that characterize Balint's syndrome. Thus, it is likely that regional hypometabolic changes seen on PET scanning are representative of the underlying regional distribution of plaques and tangles.

In evaluating (and studying) the AD patient with selective cognitive deficits, there are at least two important assumptions that need explicit discussion. One assumption is that the elegant path of tissue destruction in AD can isolate and reveal specific information processing components (Armstrong et al., 1992; Arriagada et al., 1992). The second assumption is that the progressively destructive nature of AD will systematically disassemble the cognitive architecture of the information processing component (Grafman et al., 1991).

For example, stored knowledge networks are usually viewed as relational (Nebes, 1989). That is, the "nodes" (i.e., the particular unit of information, such as a word) in such a network (i.e., the information processing component, such as a lexicon) are believed to be interconnected on the basis of some relational metric (Chertkow and Bub, 1990). In the case of a lexical network, the relational metric might be similarity in meaning, frequency of use, or category membership. Perhaps all three properties would be instantiated within a single network using three vectors.

In any case, how might damage caused by AD to that cortical network affect information accessibility? If the cortical network were spatially structured based on provinces of knowledge, then categorical deficits might be common (e.g., inability to recognize animal names but intact ability to recognize the names of tools). If the network structure contained "distributed" knowledge, then damage to a part of the network might reduce the likelihood of retrieving the least frequently used an most "weakly" stored item within the network, as its retrieval required more "evidence", i.e., greater activation of nodes (a greater sum of activated neurons) within the network. AD is uniquely able to unpeel the essential architecture of these representational networks by virtue of its slow but progressive course of damage to localized cortical regions.

A third assumption is that cognitive components topographically map onto cortical regions. As AD renders a regional network (or set of related networks) progressively more dysfunctional, then it follows that the progressive but consistent loss of accessibility to "kinds" of information should reveal the structure by which that information was stored.

Individual differences are very important in cognitive neuropsychological research and, given that AD pathophysiology may be more heterogeneous than previously suspected, the within-subject longitudinal study in AD seems superior to the cross-sectional design for the purposes of studyging a breakdown in knowledge representation. The study of patients with progressive aphasia would be particularly suited to this design (Chawluk et al., 1986; Weintraub et al., 1990); see Mesulam and Weintraub, this volume).

Another advantage heterogeneity offers the neuropsychological investigator is that the componential analysis of impaired information processing, previously neglected in AD research, is quite possible. That is, the selectivity of the pathophysiology in AD, particularly at the cortical level, can result in component-specific deficits. For example, it should be possible to identify component-specific recognition deficits (e.g., semantic versus object form agnosia) in AD patients (Martin, 1990; Saffran et al., 1990).

AD is a progressive disease which severely affects almost all cognitive functions by the time its course has run. Yet the subgroups of AD patients who display distinctive profiles of neuropsychological deficits are of sufficient size that they can be studies for their own sake (Jorm, 1985). The advantage of studying those subgroups that appear unusual is that the specificity and progression of the associated cognitive deficit(s) may uniquely reveal the successive layers of representation of a particular knowledge domain. Thus, the realization of heterogeneity in AD makes a particular subgroup of patients amenable to the kinds of studies that are crucial to understanding the distinctions in, and the structure of, knowledge representation.

Yet the heterogeneity assumption at the level of cognition implies that the best level of analysis may be at the level of the single-case. The argument here is that no two AD cases will have identical neuropathological topography and therefore identical cognitive deficits. Furthermore, individual differences in cortical folding and other normal morphological heterogeneity make every patient with a neurological disorder a potential subgroup of his/her own. We have recently published two case studies of AD patients whose selective deficits reinforce the claim that heterogeneity in AD, even at the case level, is advantageous for neuropsychological investigation.

Case Study I

Patient G. C. came to our attention after he reported he was having difficulty calculating. This retired U.S. Army General had been the president of an engineering firm when he began to experience difficulty in tabulating data, balancing his checkbook, and remembering telephone numbers. He was referred to our research group following a clinical evaluation which determined that he had probable AD. We were able to study G. C. in some detail over the subsequent two years. A detailed description of this case is available eleswhere (Grafman et al., 1989). Given that dyscalculia was his initial and outstanding cognitive deficit, we decided that a comprehensive examination and error analysis of G. C.'s number processing and calculation skills might reveal novel information about the cognitive architecture of the number and calculation procedure lexicons, as well as verify aspects of the componential cognitive models that have recently been developed to account for the varieties of dyscalculia.

We examined G. C. with both standardized and experimental tests of number processing and calculation. He was required to make judgments about magnitude, numeration, fractions, measurement, money, and time. He had to solve word problems and standard addition, subtraction, multiplication, and division problems. Other tasks required him to transcode between arabic numerals and number-words. He also had to read numbers alound, remember number sets, understand the meaning of procedural signs (e.g., +), and detect solution errors in completed problems (among other tasks).

Our longitudinal findings suggested that G. C. was experiencing an orderly dissolution of calculation and number processing ability with different dissociations apparent at different stages of decline. His number reading and writing errors (of number syntax) were qualitatively different from the errors (lexical) he made in calculation. Numerosity judgment and magnitude comparisons were intact even when G. C.'s other arithmetic knowledge and calculation abilities were grossly impaired. G. C.'s decline was first noted on more complex problems (e.g., multiplication) and only at later stages on simpler problems (e.g., addition). He was aware that aspects of his number processing and calculation performance were impaired, but he was unable to articulate why he was failing.

Many of these findings were of theoretical interest. His inability to multiply and divide (he consistently failed on *both* production and recognition tasks) in light of intact retrieval of addition and subtraction procedures indicated that such procedures were stored categorically. G. C.'s lexical errors were predominant on calculation tasks, whereas his reading and writing performance resulted in mostly syntactic errors. Thus, procedural (i.e., syntactic) rules remained relatively preserved for addition and substraction. The patient's decline in performance over time eventually affected his ability to substract. Gradually, only a few numbers were still recognized by G. C., whether in arabic or number-word forms. Even his ability to perform addition problems deteriorated so that he could only add single-digit (i.e., high frequency) numbers after two years (although no particular single-digit numbers were spared; e.g., the digits 0–4).

These data, collected from an AD patient, helped in articulating a cognitive model of number and calculation procedure representation. They suggested that numbers and computational facts are stored in a lexical-like network. The all-or-none loss of calculation procedures indicated that procedures are principally stored categorically. More importantly for this chapter, a patient with AD had a consistent decline in a relatively specific domain that led to several new hypotheses regarding the representation of knowledge within that domain. Although this patient was globally demented by our last evaluation, the relative selectivity of his deficit in the early stages of his disease, in conjunction with the effect his progressive decline had on the structure of domain-specific information, allowed him to contribute significantly to current cognitive neuropsychological knowledge. Of course, many other examples now exist that show the usefulness of longitudinally studying patients whose disorder has a progressive course. However, AD patients who remain cognitively stable even for a few months, but have selective deficits, can also help contribute to knowledge about basic brain-behavior relationships.

Case Study II

Autotopagnosia is an inability to locate body parts on verbal command. It does not appear as an isolated disorder; rather it is usually one of a cluster of deficits that can include aphasia, apraxia, neglect, and motor control disorders. There have been two divergent views of the cause of autotopagnosia. One view suggests that autotopagnosia reflects an impaired spatial representation of the body schema. The other view claims that autotopagnosia reflects a more basic deficit in analyzing part-whole relationships. We recently identified a case that appeared to demonstrate a relatively selective body schema deficit. This patients, with probable AD, elegantly demonstrated that a body schema deficit could be observed independently of spatial location problems.

The details of this case are available in a recent publication (Sirigu et al., 1991). In brief, the patient was evaluated by us about three years after the onset of her symptoms. She came to our attention because a ward nurse noticed that she was having exceptional difficulty in getting dressed in the morning because of an inability to match her body parts with the correct piece or part of clothing. On a formal evaluation, the patient was impaired in localizing body parts on herself, the examiner, or a doll *to verbal command*. This deficit was most severe when she had to point to her own body. Nonverbal instructions were also of little use. Curiously, the patient was able to name body parts quite accurately. Most of her pointing errors were aimed at body parts that were adjacent to the target body part. Other experiments were performed to confirm what appeared to be a selective deficit in accessing body schema knowledge. Perhaps the most convincing experiment we conducted involved the placing of objects on the examiner's body and on the body of the patient. Incredibly, the patient was able to accurately point to object targets on herself or the examiner that were pinned to body parts that earlier, or later, in the same session she was unable to point to accurately. Unfortunately, the patient was unable to learn to use the object to mediate her pointing to the body part even though she was able to accurately remember the location of the objects on her body for several days after the experiments were completed.

The results of this case study motivated us to develop a componential model of body "knowledge" that specified our patient's deficit at the level of visual-spatial/structural representations of the body, whereas her semantic representations of the body and its parts were intact, as was her three-dimensional body-reference system, given her accurate object pointing.

These two carefully selected probable AD patients made significant contributions to models of number processing/calculation and body knowledge representation because of the uniqueness of their cognitive deficits. This uniqueness reflects the heterogeneity of AD at the single-case level.

Discussion

The evidence from both case and group studies demonstrates that AD expresses itself heterogeneously on both a cognitive and pathophysiological level (Bondareff et al., 1987; Van Hoesen and Hyman, 1990). Furthermore, this clinical phenomena is of sufficient frequency that its study will benefit the construction of models of various cognitive components and their representational architecture. Moreover, it appears that this neuropsychological heterogeneity neatly maps onto the underlying pathophysiologic process at the cortical level (Hof et al., 1989).

This heterogeneity in AD demands a broad-based clinical neuropsychological approach to identify appropriate subgroups and candidates for detailed research studies. It also is a clear argument for the use of AD patients in single-case and subgroup studies designed to formulate more precise brain-behavior relationships. It remains unclear whether pharmacologic and other intervention trials should utilize distinct subgroups of AD patients to maximize the liklihood of observing changes in a few cognitive domains. Although it is clear that most drug trials target changes on so-called episodic or declarative memory measures that reflect the most common disorder in AD, trials tailored towards remediating an outstanding, but selective, deficit such as a progressive visuospatial disorder should be considered (Saffran et al., 1990; Cronin-Golomb et al., 1991a, b).

What is not yet clear is whether this neurophysological and pathophysiological heterogeneity reflects distinct underlying biological causes or is merely the multivariate expression of a single underlying disease process. There are, of course, other diseases besides AD that lead to a progressive dementia, including frontal and Pick's dementias (and perhaps some or all cases of progressive aphasia) which may only be distinguishable at autopsy.

For the AD patient, this heterogeneity of neuropsychological deficit, in combination with the progressive nature of the deficit, leads to the disappearance of conceptually driven knowledge, such as the meaning of a word. Data-driven knowledge, such as the ability to simply read a word, appears relatively preserved, even during the later stages of AD. This loss of semantic or conceptually driven knowledge is progressive but slow. The patient may be aware of his or her disappearing knowledge store to some degree but cannot easily compensate for its loss. The argument that there is a disappearance of knowledge as opposed to an access problem is based upon numerous studies of impaired semantic knowledge in AD patients, as well as the fact that the AD pathophysiological process destroys the integrity of those cortical networks which presumably subserve the "lost" knowledge (Hyman et al., 1990).

This pathophysiological process reduces the number of functioning cells within a regional cortical networks as well as degrading the inter-regional communication and binding process. AD is a progressive disease and an ever-increasing number of cells become dysfunctional over time. To interpret the impact of this kind of pathological process on cognition, it is necessary to assume a certain kind of representational architecture for cognitive processes, although the specifics of the relational bonds within the architecture are not absolutely relevant for this particular argument. The representational architecture does need to be a distributed representational network that would have various entries activated on the principal basis of strength and pattern of information. In this scenerio, the fewer cells available for activation within a regional cognitive network, the less likely that items more weakly represented within the network (and therefore requiring a greater amount of activation which would be dependent upon a greater participation of neurons within the network) would be activated to a level that would produce a behavioral effect (e.g., recognition, priming, etc.). This kind of deficit I view as a "storage" problem, as opposed to an "access" problem in which the information could be sufficiently activated for some behavioral purposes (consistent implicit or occasional explicit recognition) but not others, such as consistent conscious recognition. Thus, in the two cases I described above, it is likely that a disappearance of knowledge regarding calculation procedures and numbers as well as the body schema contributed to their deficits.

Are there other types of neuropsychological investigations that could benefit from the heterogeneity of the cognitive disorders in these patients? Studies of attention (Sahakian et al., 1990) and consciousness (Lopez et al., 1991) would be two prime candidates that have been relatively neglected in the study of AD patients. Some views of consciousness argue that it is an epiphenomenon composed of the currently activated representational networks (both data and conceptually driven). Therefore, if networks become inoperative due to AD, then a systematic degradation or distortion of consciousness should occur. AD patients would then be expected to have different kinds of "combinatorial consciousness" depending on which representational domains were preserved and which were lost. Attention has been viewed as being domain-specific and also having qualities that cut across domains. AD would be an ideal disorder in which to address these two views since it results in both generalized (e.g., memory) and domain-specific (e.g., aphasia) impairments.

In conclusion, the heterogeneous disappearance of knowledge in AD is a frequent occurrence at both the group and individual case levels. This neuropsychological heterogeneity expresses itself by componential dissociations within the framework of an information processing model and maps onto pathophysiologic topography. The selectivity of the cognitive deficits in AD along with their inalterable progression suggests that studies designed to gain a better understanding of the cognitive architecture of the affected components can make a valuable contribution to cognitive science. Surely the recognition of heterogeneity in AD will increase the usefulness of AD patients as subjects in neuropsychological studies, if not lead to a better understanding of the biological mechanism(s) by which AD expresses itself.

References

Armstrong RA, Myers D, Smith CUM, Cairns N, Luthert PJ (1992) The spatial pattern of senile plaques, neurofibrillary tangles and A4 deposits in Alzheimer's disease. Neurosci Res Com 10:27–33

Arriagada PV, Growdon JH, Hodley-White ET, Hyman BT (1992) Neurofibrillary tangles but not senile plaques parallel duration and severity of Alzheimer's disease. Neurology 42:631–639

Bondareff W, Mountjoy CQ, Roth M, Rossor MN, Iversen LL, Reynolds GP (1987) Age and histopathologic heterogeneity in Alzheimer's disease. Arch Gen Psychiat 44:412–417

Celsis P, Agniel A, Puel M, Rascol A, Marc-Vergnes JP (1987) Focal cerebral hypoperfusion and selective cognitive deficit in dementia of the Alzheimer type. J Neurol Neurosurg Psychiatr 50:1602–1612

Chawluk JB, Mesulam M-M, Hurtig H, Kushner M, Weintraub S, Saykin A, Rubin N, Alavi A, Reivich M (1986) Slowly progressive aphasia without generalized dementia: studies with positron emission tomography. Ann Neurol, 19:68–74

Chertkow H, Bub D (1990) Semantic memory loss in dementia of Alzheimer's type: what do various measures measure? Brain, 113:397–417

Cronin-Golomb A, Corkin S, Rizzo JF, Cohen J, Growdon JH, Banks KS (1991a) Visual dysfunction in Alzheimer's disease: relation to normal aging. Ann Neurol 29:41–52

Cronin-Golomb A, Rizzo JF, Corkin S, Growdon JH (1991b) Visual function in Alzheimer's disease and normal aging. In: Growdon JH, Corkin S, Ritter-Walker E, Wurtman RJ (eds) Aging and Alzheimer's disease: sensory systems, neuronal growth, and neuronal metabolism. The New York Academy of Sciences, New York, pp 28–35

Grafman J, Kampen D, Rosenberg J, Salazar AM, Boller F (1989) The progressive breakdown of number processing and calculation ability: a case study. Cortex, 25:121–133

Grafman J, Thompson K, Weingartner H, Martinez R, Lawlor BA, Sunderland T (1991) Script generation as an indicator of knowledge representation in patients with Alzheimer's disease. Brain Lang, 40:344–358

Haxby J (1990) Cognitive deficits and local metabolic changes in dementia of the Alzheimer type. In: Rapoport SR, Petit H, Leys D, Christen Y (eds) Imaging, cerebral topography, and Alzheimer's disease. Springer-Verlag, Berlin, pp 109–120

Hof PR, Bouras C, Constantinidis J, Morrison JH (1989) Balint's syndrome in Alzheimer's disease: specific disruption of the occipito-parietal visual pathway. Brain Res 493:368–375

Hyman BT, Van Hoesen GW, Damasio AR (1990) Memory-related neural systems in Alzheimer's disease: an anatomic study. Neurology 40:1721–1730

Jorm AF (1985) Subtypes of Alzheimer's dementia: a conceptual analysis and critical review: Psychol Med 15:543–553

Kobayashi K, Kurachi M, Gyoubu T, Fukutani Y, Inao G, Nakamura I, Yamaguchi N (1990) Progressive dysphasia dementia with localized cerebral atrophy: report of an autopsy. Clin Neuropathol 9:254–261

Lopez OL, Becker JT, Brenner RP, Rosen J, Bajulaige OI, Reynolds CF (1991) Alzheimer's disease with delusions and hallucinations: neuropsychological and electroencephalographic correlates. Neurology 41:906–912

Martin A (1987) Representation of semantic and spatial knowledge in Alzheimer's patients: implications for models of preserved learning in amnesia. J Clin Exp Neurophsychol 9:191–224

Martin A (1990) Neuropsychology of Alzheimer's Disease: The Case for Subgroups. In: Schwartz MF (Ed) Modular deficits in Alzheimer-type dementia. Bradford Book, The MIT Press, Cambridge, pp 143–176

Martin A, Brouwers P, Lalonde F, Cox C, Teleska P, Fedio P, Foster NL, Chase TN (1986) Towards a behavioral typology of Alzheimer's patients. J Clin Exp Neuropsychol 8:594–610

McKhann G, Drachman D, Folstein M, Katzman R, Price D, Stadlan EM (1984) Clinical diagnosis of Alzheimer's disease: Report of the NINCDS-ADRDA work group under the auspices of Department of Health and Human Services Task Force on Alzheimer's Disease. Neurology 34:939–944

Morrison JH, Hof PR, Bouras C (1991) An anatomic substrate for visual disconnection in Alzheimer's disease. In: Growdon JH, Corkin S, Ritter-Wolker E, Wurtman RJ (eds) Aging and Alzheimer's disease. The New York Academy of Sciences, New York, pp 36–43

Nebes R (1989) Semantic memory in Alzheimer's disease. Psych Bull 106:377–394

Poeck K, Luzzatti C (1988) Slowly progressive aphasia in three patients. Brain 111:151–169

Pogacar S, Williams RS (1984) Alzheimer's disease presenting as slowly progressive aphasia. RI Med J 67:181–185

Saffran EM, Fitzpatric-DeSalme EJ, Coslett HB (1990) Visual disturbances in dementia. In: Schwartz MF (Ed) Modular deficits in Alzheimer-type dementia. Bradford Book, The MIT Press, Cambridge, pp 297–328

Sahakian BJ, Downes JJ, Eagger S, Evenden JL, Lery R, Philpot MP, Roberts AC, Robbins TW (1990) Sparing of attentional relative to mnemonic function in a subgroup of patients with dementia of the Alzheimer type. Neuropsychology 28:1197–1213

Schwartz MF (ed) (1990) Modular deficits in Alzheimer-type dementia. Issues in the biology of language and cognition. Bradford Book, The MIT Press, Cambridge pp 1–346

Schwartz MF, Chawluk JB (1990) Deterioration of language in progressive aphasia: a case study. In: Schwartz MF (ed) Modular deficits in Alzheimer-type dementia. Bradford Book, The MIT Press, Cambridge, pp 245–296

Sirigu A, Grafman J, Bressler K, Sunderland T (1991) Multiple representations contribute to body knowledge processing. Brain 114:629–642

Van Hoesen GW, Damasio AR (1987) Neural correlates of cognitive impairment in Alzheimer's disease. In: Plum F (ed) Higher functions of the nervous system: the handbook of physiology. Williams and Wilkins, Baltimore, pp 871–898

Van Hoesen GW, Hyman BT (1990) Hippocampal formation: anatomy and the patterns of pathology in Alzheimer's disease. In: Storm-Mathisen J, Zimmer J, Ottersen OP (eds) Progress in Brain Research. Vol 83. Elsevier, Amsterdam, pp 445–457

Weintraub S, Rubin NP, Mesulam M-M (1990) Primary progressive aphasia: longitudinal course, neuropsychological profile, and language features. Arch Neurol 47:1329–1335

Neuropsychological Aspects of Alzheimer's Disease: Evidence for Inter- and Intra-Function Heterogeneity

Y. Joanette, B. Ska, A. Poissant, and *R. Béland*

Summary

The goal of the present chapter is to provide an overview of the question of the heterogeneity of neuropsychological manifestations in Alzheimer's disease (AD). The classical views, which contend that neuropsychological manifestations in AD are homogeneous, are reported and discussed. Among other things, these classical views are felt to be limited either by the restricted nature of the test batteries used or by their intrinsic non-specificity. The results of recent group studies and multiple single-case studies are taken as strongly indicative of the presence of heterogeneity, both between distinct cognitive functions *and* between a given cognitive function's subcomponents. The conditions are such that different patients can exhibit reverse patterns of cognitive impairments at both levels, i.e, inter- and intrafunctions. The presence of this heterogeneity cannot be solely linked with the known heterogeneity in AD itself (e.g., distribution of the neuropathological alterations) but could also reflect inter-individual differences in brain organization for cognition, or suspected changes with age of this organization, or even the exacerbation of heterogeneity of cognitive functioning in normal aging itself. Despite the presence of such confounding factors, it is hoped that neuropsychologically defined subgroups of AD may overlap with other biologically defined subgroups. From a practical point of view, the need to use a detailed and theoretically motivated cognitive procedure in any study of AD partly or totally based upon neuropsychological descriptors is stressed in order to overcome the confusion that could be generated by the presence of such heterogeneity.

Introduction

From a clinical point of view, Alzheimer's disease (AD) is a behavioural condition before it is a neurobiological condition. Until it is possible to determine biological markers of the disease, AD patients will be identified on the basis of the existence of gradual changes in personality and in cognitive functioning. As the former are difficult to evaluate and not easy to quantify, the latter has become the basis for the diagnosis of AD. Thus, neuropsychological signs constitute the essence of the positive inclusion criteria in many diagnostic approaches meant to provide, with a distinct level of confidence, a pre-mortem diagnosis of putative AD (e.g., McKhann et al., 1984). At the same time, most of the research projects done on the effects of experimental drugs are based

F. Boller et al. (Eds.)
Heterogeneity of Alzheimer's Disease
© Springer-Verlag Berlin Heidelberg 1992

upon an evaluation of changes in neuropsychological abilities to provide support for the possible efficacy of given molecules (Gauthier et al., 1991). The cognitive functioning of AD patients is thus important not only for patient identification; it also serves as a basis for much other research done from biological, epidemiological, neurochemical, genetic and neuropathological perspectives. However, it is becoming more and more obvious that AD does not represent a unique, homogeneous at pathological state at any of these levels. It is, therefore, of the upmost importance to consider the fact that the neuropsychological manifestations of AD in the early stages of the disease also do not appear to be homogeneous. It is the purpose of this chapter to provide a brief overview of the literature on this topic and to show that, in AD, the heterogeneity of the neuropsychological manifestations is probably greater than expected, not only when comparing different cognitive functions but also when considering the sub-components of a given cognitive function.

The degree to which neuropsychological manifestations of AD have been considered homogeneous or heterogenous should be linked with the degree of refinement used to describe these neuropsychological signs. As Martin (1990) reminds the case described by Alzheimer (1907) himself was first perceived as a personality change. Only later was Alzheimer struck by the fact that memory and other cognitive functions were also deteriorating. This is not surprising since, at the turn of the century, neuropsychology was yet to be introduced as a field and that, consequently, the available conceptual and methodological tools for evaluating cognitive functioning were very limited. Years later, the position defended by the Geneva school is probably attributable to the same limitations. Indeed, this school proposed (e.g., Richard and Constantinidis, 1970) that neuropsychological manifestations of AD were to be regarded as a homogeneous impairment of language, perceptual abilities and gestural abilities, the so-called aphaso-agnoso-apractic syndrome. Thus, it was claimed that all aspects of cognition had to be affected equally at a given point in the patient's evolution. If one cognitive function was affected at a given level, it was predicted that other cognitive functions would be affected at the same level at the same time (Richard and Constantinids, 1970). A somewhat similar point of view is still defended by authors using classical neuropsychometric approaches. For example, Hom (1992) reported the presence of a single homogeneous pattern of neuropsychological impairment in AD patients using the Halsted-Reitan Neuropsychological Test Battery for Adults, along with complementary procedures (Reitan and Davison, 1974). According to Hom (1992), all measures of "generalized neuropsychological functions" are affected in AD patients along with nearly all other "neuropsychological functions."

However, it has become obvious to anyone in cognitive neuropsychology that such a homogeneous conception of neuropsychological manifestations of AD is untenable. The position defended by the Geneva school may reflect the fact that the patients they examined were already at more severe stages of the disease, thus preventing the appreciation of inter-patient differences, or with the fact that neuropsychological descriptors used in those studies were still very general and had not yet benefitted from the extraordinary input of cognitive psychology that would come later. On the other hand, a neuropsychometric approach such as the one Hom (1992) uses is also limited by the facts that a) the concept of "generalized neuropsychological functions" is by definition general, thus unsurprisingly yields a deficit, whatever the task used to measure it; and b) the different neuropsychological functions according to this approach are defined by reference to the task proposed rather than an explicit model of normal cognition. In fact, as we shall see in the following paragraphs, since the early, 1970s, many case studies and group studies using specific descriptors have provided evidence against the postulated homogeneity of neuropsychological manifestations in AD.

The birth of cognitive heterogeneity

Clinical experience clearly shows that although all AD patients tend to look the same from a cognitive standpoint at later stages of the disease, the array of cognitive impairments can be very different in the early and middle stages of the disease (Schwartz, 1990). Of course, such heterogeneity cannot be appreciated through the use of gross evaluation of cognitive functioning, such as the use of brief bedside procedure of the Mini Mental State Examination type (Folstein et al., 1975), Unfortunately, these procedures do not allow us to adequately appreciate all the aspects of the impaired cognitive functioning in a given patient. In fact, most of these brief procedures include only limited aspects of cognitive functioning (gestural abilities are only rarely included). Moreover, the sub-headings in these brief procedures are illusory most of the time, since most of the tasks require language for understanding the required execution, thus biasing towards linguistic abilities any measure taken.

For these reasons, many neurologists and epidemiologists have overlooked, in the past, the presence of heterogeneity in the early and middle stages of the disease. However, a number of better documented case reports have been a source of inspiration for many neuropsychologists. One of the frequently cited reports of a case of autopsy-confirmed AD with a non-classical presentation is that of Crystal et al. (1981). This was the case of a patient whose neuropsychological impairments were biased in favor of visuo-spatial abilities. Thus, in the presence of relatively preserved linguistic skills, this AD patient was performing particularly badly on visuospatial tasks. It was later confirmed that the neuropathological alterations were predominant over the right hemisphere, and therefore in accordance with the pre-mortem imbalance between the impairments of language and visuo-spatial abilities. Similar results were reported by other authors using regional cerebral blood flow or PET scans to appreciate, in vivo, the relative degree of hypometabolism in each hemisphere (Celsis et al., 1987). But the functional organization of cognition in the brain is certainly not limited to a left-right opposition. The secular focal lesion literature has clearly demonstrated that patients with very similar but slightly different lesions can exhibit very different cognitive impairment patterns and sometimes, in fact, reversed patterns. This can be seen either when comparing the relative impairment of different cognitive functions (e.g., language versus memory) or when looking at the sub-components of a given function (e.g., syntactical abilities versus the processing of words). Not surprisingly, the literature has now come up with plenty of examples of different patterns of cognitive impairments in AD. The following summarizes the results of some of the most cited group studies.

Group studies and the case for subgroups of AD patients

Since the 1980s, a number of group studies have been reported in the literature showing the existence of subgroups of AD patients determined on the basis of their cognitive impairment profiles. One of these studies is that of Martin et al. (1986). Despite the limited character of the neuropsychological protocol used, these authors showed that a large proportion (40%) of early dementia of the Alzheimer type (DAT) patients (McKhann et al., 1984) had a cognitive impairment which did not affect all functions equally. Hence, of the 42 patients examined, only 25 (60%) had an impairment which looked quite even across the different cognitive functions examined. Nine DAT patients exhibited more language impairments whereas eight other patients showed a somewhat reversed pattern. Quite similar data were reported by Neary et al. (1986), though based on a smaller number of patients examined. Thus, the same proportion of AD patients (11 of 18, or 61%) showed what the Geneva school referred to as an aphaso-apracto-agnosic syndrome, or a quite similar impairment of most cognitive functions. In three patients (17%), the memory impairment was accompanied by some language and visuo-constructive deficits, whereas in two patients (11%), visuo-constructive deficits appeared to predominate. Finally, in two other patients (11%), memory deficits were largely dominating.

A much larger group of DAT patients was looked at with similar goals by Becker et al. (1988). These authors examned 86 patients with a DAT diagnosis, many of them autopsy-confirmed AD. Despite the limited nature of the neuropsychological protocol, the results were very similar to those reported by Martin et al. (1986). In fact, nearly one of five DAT patients exhibited a severe impairment of one given cognitive function. In many cases, the impairment pattern was reversed, thus suggesting the existence of dissociatons.

The importance of these group studies is obvious. They have awakened researchers in the field of neuropsychology to the existence of possible subgroups of AD patients which could correspond to etiologically distinct subtypes of AD (Jorm, 1985). However, these studies are still gross from a neuropsychological point of view. Indeed, most of them are based on a neuropsychological protocol which is made up of a very limited number of tasks, each of them felt to be able to measure one given cognitive function. But cognitive functions are complex by themselves and are made up of many cognitive sub-components. Thus, not taking into account all the known cognitive functions *and* their sub-components could resemble trying to find the genetic characteristics of AD while using only half a dozen probe corresponding to an equal number of loci on a randomly chosen gene. Thus, it is necessary to use all the possibilities offered by modern cognitive neuropsychology to describe comprehensively the possible existence in AD patients of such heterogeneity in the relative impairment of cognitive functions, or of their sub-components. Some preliminary data are provided below.

Inter- and intra-cognitive functions heterogeneity: the multiple single-case approach

As pointed out by Martin (1990), the only way to ascertain the existence of neuropsychologically determined subgroups in AD is to demonstrate the existence of double dissociations between single subjects and to confirm that these double dissociations are indeed representative of a given cluster of AD patients. And the only way that double dissociations can possibly be demonstrated is through the use of a multiple single-subject paradigm (Caramazza, 1986).

Using such an approach, Joanette and colleagues (1989 and in preparation) presented data that suggest the existence of contrastive patterns of cognitive impairments in a group of patients with DAT. Eleven early-stage DAT patients were submitted to a thorough neuropsychological examination meant to evaluate most of the sub-components of language, memory and gestural as well as perceptual abilities. All in all, the protocol required more than 12 hours of testing. Each patient's performance on each task was compared with that of a group of control subjects matched for age, sex and level of education. Results showed that only a minority of DAT patients evidenced a somewhat homogeneous impairment of all cognitive functions. Indeed, only four patients (36%) were more or less equally affected on all cognitive functions, despite the fact that, at this point, performance on sub-components was not considered independently. In four other patients (36%), the relative impairment related to each cognitive function was somewhat unequal. However, in the remaining three subjects, the dissociations were much more important. Among those subjects, some had quite contrastive patterns. Thus, whereas one patient had an impairment of language in the presence of preserved perceptual abilities, another patient had the reverse pattern, namely impaired perceptual abilities along with intact linguistic skills. If the results of these studies are confirmed, then it could be maintained that only a minority of DAT patients present themselves with a somewhat homogeneous impairment of all cognitive functions. The majority of patients appear to show contrastive patterns which, in some cases, can even result in apparent dissociations. However, only large-scale, single-case studies coupled with cluster-seeking group studies will allow us to see if those contrastive patterns are unique to each subject or if there are cognitive impairment patterns that can be found among subgroups of DAT patients.

Another level which is even less explored is the comparison between the relative impairments of given cognitive function subcomponents. Indeed, nearly all of the studies looking at neuropsychological heterogeneity in AD have focused on a comparison *between* the relative impairment of a given set of cognitive functions. As mentioned before, most of previous studies neuropsychological evaluations were neither well constructed nor complete enough to allow a systematic comparison between a given cognitive functions's sub-components. In a recent study, Ska et al. (1990, submitted for publication) have looked at some language sub-components in a systematic manner.

The classical theory regarding the relative impairment of language sub-components in AD refers to a homogeneous, progressive pattern. It is still thought that AD first affects the semantic processing of words, then the ability to construct sentences through syntactic abilities, and finally the ability to plan and organize the sounds of language through phonology (Cardebat et al., 1991), However, careful analysis of each of thes three levels of abilities in a group of early-stage DAT patients did not confirm this theory. Analyzing the respective semantic, syntactic and phonological abilities of 12 DAT patients compared to those of a group of normal aging patients, matched for age, sex and level of education, Ska et al. (1990) found that only half of the subjects (7 or 58%) had performance compatible with this classical theory. Most of the other DAT patients had contrastive patterns, according to which, for example, syntactical and phonological abilities could be impaired in the absence of any gross impairment of semantic abilities. This result remains to be confirmed in a larger group of subjects, in order to seek recurrent patterns of impairments of language sub-components that could indicate the existence of subgroups of AD patients determined by profiles of impairments of subcomponents of language function. It also remains to be seen if the same could hold for other cognitive functions and their sub-components. But these preliminary results certainly raise the question of the possible existence of subgroups of AD patients determined not only by some inter-cognitive function distinctive profile, but also by some intra-cognitive function patterns of impairments. Such a perspective does not simplify the quest for cognitively determined subgroups of AD patients, but it certainly indicates the road to follow to identify such subgroups.

When such a quest is fulfilled then the real questions will emerge. Indeed, the ultimate question will be to identify the underlying determinants for such neuropsychologically determined subgroups in AD. And the reasons might not be as simple as they appear to be. The following section discusses this aspect of the question.

Neuropsychological heterogeneity: more than a mere reflection of neuropathological heterogeneity?

Many factors, only some of them linked with the progression of the disease, could account for the presence of neuropsychologically determined subgroups in AD. The first of these factors is obvious to readers of this book and is linked to the otherwise present heterogeneity of the neuropathological alterations in the disease (see Donnet et al., 1991, as well as other contributions in this book). It is well known that, despite some relative regularity in the distribution of the neuropathologial alterations and their progression with the disease, senile plaques and neurofibrillary tangles are not found at the exact same location from one patient to another. Not only can the relative impairment of each of the two hemispheres be different, but the exact location on the cortex of these alterations can vary. If these findings are confirmed, and it subgroups of AD patients can be identified on the basis of some neuropathological profiles, then these subgroups could possibly overlap with neuropsychologically determined subgroups.

The study of focal brain damage has shown that there are some brain-behaviour regularities. The lesion of a given portion of the cortex can be correlated with the impairment of a given set of sub-components of one or more cognitive functions. However, the same literature also tell us that this regularity is, at most, loose, and that one should not expect too much from it (Basso et al., 1985). Thus, there might be some confounding factors that could prevent us from obtaining a nice correspondence between neuropsychologically and neuropathologically determined subgroups of AD patients.

The first of the possible confounding factors emanates, as alluded to before, from the focal brain lesion literature in neuropsychology. Since the advent of modern static and dynamic brain-imaging techniques (e.g., CT and MRI scans as well as PET scans), the classical teaching with regard to brain-cognition relationships has been confronted with unexpected data. The first of these data has been the extent to which a given lesion can express itself very differently in distinct individuals. Thus, a lesion of the left supramarginalis gyrus does not always actualize itself through a conduction aphasia. The resulting neuropsychological impairments can differ quite amazingly from one patient to another. It is known that some intrinsic (e.g., sex, personal, as well as familial handedness) as well as extrinsic (eg., nature of spoken and written language, knowledge of second language, level of education) factors can contribute to such differences. Be that as it may, patients who are developing AD are certainly no more homogeneous in their pre-morbid brain's functional organization than patients who have been studied following focal brain damage. The result is that even if all AD patients exhibited the exact same pattern of neuropathological degeneration (and we have seen that this is not the case) the neuropsychological manifestations could differ according to these intrinsic and extrinsic factors that determine a given individuals specific brain organization for cognition.

But there is more to it. Indeed, above and beyond these differences, it is also now suspected, at least for language, that a given individuals brain functional organization may change with age, within adulthood (see Joanette et al., 1983, for a review). Dynamic models proposing a constant evolution of the functional organization of the brain have been proposed (Goldberg and Costa,, 1981; Hanlon, 1991). These models were proposed, among other reasons, to explain why given types of aphasia are age-associated. For instance, more than a dozen large-scale studies have now confirmed that the mean age of Broca's aphasics is some 10 years less than the man age of Wernicke's aphasics, without any change in the topographic distribution of the responsible brain lesions. If that piece of knowledge is correct, then the effects of a degenerative condition such as AD might be different according to the age of the patient at onset. Along with the inter-individual differences noted earlier, this finding could seriously endangered the search for some overlap between neuropsychologically and neuropathologically determined subgroups of AD.

Finally, another confounding factor could be normal aging itself. Indeed, all of the studies looking at the possible existence of neuropsychologically determined subgroups of AD patients have been testing patients in the early stages of the disease. This is normal since, with time, cognitive functioning is so affected in AD that any test batteries usually yield floor-effect performance. But the fact that most of the evidence comes from a point in time when the patient's performance is not immensely different from those of normal-aged controls raises the question of the influence of normal aging on the resulting data. One possible confounding factor is the homogeneous or heterogeneous nature of normal aging itself. This question has received surpringly little attention in the past. In a study done a few years ago, Valdois et al. (1990) clearly showed that normal aging is far from homogeneous from a neuropsychological point of view. Using a comprehensive neuropsychological battery with some 70 medically confirmed normal subjects, these authors showed that normal-aged subjects can be distinguished in at least two aspects. The first one is a performance factor, which simply means that some subjects are globally better than others. But the second factor was a qualitative one. Particularly among those subjects who performed least well – despite the fact that they were still largely within the limit of normality – the existence of contrastive patterns of cognitive abilities could be demonstrated. In other words, even before AD strikes into a population of normal-aged subjects, a non-trivial proportion of these have distinct cognitive patterns that, in some cases, can be the reverse of their neighbour's cognitive patterns. One possibility is that this condition could be exacerbated with the advent of an incoming AD process and could, again, contribute to the existence of distinctive patterns of cognitive impairments. This contribution, if it is confirmed, could represent another undesired, but definitely present, confounding factor.

Conclusion

The existence of heterogeneity in the neuropsychologial manifestations of AD is beyond doubt. In fact, a contrary finding would have been surprising, given the complexity of the disease itself and the even greater complexity of the brain-behavior relationship. It is now well known that this heterogeneity is to be found both between different cognitive functions *and* within the sub-components of a given cognitive function. The extent to which this heterogeneity can be demonstrated is frequently linked with the degree to which the neuropsychological descriptors are sufficiently precise and theoretically motivated. In most non-neuropsychological studies (e.g., neuropathological, epidemiological, genetic. clinical trials), the neuropsychological procedures used are, at most, gross and do not allow us, to adequately appreciate the cognitive functioning of the patients. Despite the fact that this heterogeneity is definitely present in AD, it is not clear that all of it should be attributed to AD itself. It has been argued that part of this heterogeneity may correspond to the expression of inter-individual differences in brain organization for cognition under the influence of intrinsic and extrinsic factors, along with the influence of age. Moreover, whatever the precise organization of a given individual, it has also been stressed that there are inter-individual differences in the cognitive abilities of normal-aged subjects than can be such that contrastive patterns of functioning can be found, even within the limits of normality. The latter could thus be amplified by the unfortunate influence of AD in the early stages of the disease.

Despite all this, it is to be hoped that well constructed studies will be able to disentangle all these factors and to combine the neuropsychologically based information regarding heterogeneity in AD with that issuing from other approaches to the disease, namely epidemiological, neurochemical, genetic and neuropathological. Only to the extent that the level of sophistication is equivalent in all of those approaches will there be some chance that the veil still covering this disease might be someday raised.

Acknowledgments. This work was made possible through the support of Program Grant PG-28 of the Conseil de la recherche médicale du Canada (C.R.M.C.) as well as by a grant from the Alzheimer Society of Canada to the first author. R. B. is Chercheur-boursier of the Fonds de la recherche en santé du Québec. Y. J. is Scientist of the C.R.M.C.

References

Alzheimer A (1907) A peculiar disease of the cerebral cortex (National Library of Medicine trans). Allgemeine Zeitschrift Psychiatr 64:146–158

Basso A, Lecours AR, Moraschinie S, Vanier M (1985) Anatomoclinical correlations of the aphasias defined through computerized tomography: exceptions. Brain Lang 26:201–229

Becker JT, Huff FJ, Nebes RD, Holland A, Boller F (1988) Neuropsychological function in Alzheimer's disease: Pattern of impairment and rate of progression. Arch Neurol 45:263–268

Caramazza A (1986) On drawing inferences about the structure of normal cognitive systems from the analysis of patterns of impaired performance: The case for single-patient studies. Brain Cogn 5:565–582

Cardebat D, Démonet JF, Puel M, Nespoulous JL, Rascol A (1991) Langage et démences. In: Habib M, Joanette Y, Puel M (eds) Démences et syndromes démentiels: Approche neuropsychologique. Masson & Edisem, Paris & Montréal, pp:153–164

Celsis P, Agniel A, Rascol A, Marc-Vergnes JP (1987) Focal cerebral hypoperfusion and selective cognitive deficit in dementia of the Alzheimer type. J Neurol Neurosurg Psychiatr 50:1602–1612

Crystal HA, Horoupian DS, Katzman R, Jotkowitz S (1981) Biopsy-proved Alzheimer disease presenting as right parietal lobe syndrome. Ann Neurol 12:186–188

Donnet A, Foncin JF, Habib M (1991) Démence et vieillissemnet cérébral: Evolution des concepts de l'antiquité à nos jours. In: Habib M, Joanette Y, Puel M (eds) Démences et syndromes démentiels: Approache neuropsychologique. Masson & Edisem, Paris & Montréal, pp 1–3

Folstein MF, Folstein SE, McHugh PR (1975) Mini mental state: a practical method for grading the cognitive state of patients for the clinician. J Psychiatr Res 12:189–198

Gauthier S, Quirion R, Leblanc R, Bouchard R, Gauthier L (1991) Thérapeutiques interventionnistes de la maladie d'Alzheimer. In: Habib M, Joanette Y, Puel M (eds) Démences et syndromes démenticls: Approche neuropschologique. Masson & Edisem, Paris & Montréal, pp 271–282

Goldberg E, Costa LD (1981) Hemisphere differences in the acquisition and use of descriptive systems. Brain Lang 14:144–173

Hanlon RE (ed) (1991) Cognitive microgenesis. A neuropsychological perspective. Springer, Berlin, Heidelberg, New York

Hom J (1992) General and specific cognitive dysfunctions in patients with Alzheimer's disease. Arch Clin Neuropsychol 7:121–133

Joanette Y, Poissant A, Valdois S (1989) Neuropsychological dissociations in dementia of the Alzheimer type: a multiple single case study. J Clin Exp Neuropsychol 11:91

Joanette Y, Ali-Chérif A, Delpuech F, Habib M, Pellissier JF, Poncet M (1983) Evolution de la séméiologie aphasique avec l'âge. Discussion á propos d'une observation anatomo-clinique. Rev Neurol (Paris) 139:657–664

Jorm A (1985) Subtypes of Alzheimer dementia: a conceptual analysis and critical review. Psychol Med 15:543–553

Martin A (1990) Neuropsychology of Alzheimer's disease: the case for subgroups. In: Schwartz MF (ed) Modular deficits in Alzheimer-type dementia. MIT Press, Cambridge, pp 143–175

Martin A, Brouwers P, Lalonde F, Cox C, Teleska P, Fedio P, Foster NL, Chase TN (1986) Toward a behavioral typology of Alzheimer's patients. J Clin Exp Neuropsychol 8:594–610

McKhann G, Drachman D, Folstein M, Katzman R, Price D, Stadlan EM (1984) Clinical diagnosis of Alzheimer's disease: Report of the NINCDS-ADRDA work group under the auspices of Department of Health and Human Services task force on Alzheimer's disease. Neurology 34:939–944

Neary D, Snowden JS, Bowen DM, Sims NR, Mann D, Benton JS,Northen B, Yates P, Avison D (1986) Neuropsychological syndromes in presenile dementia due to cerebral atrophy. J Neurol Neurosurg Neuropsychiat 49:163–174

Reitan RM, Davison LA (eds) (1974) Clinical neuropsychology: current status and application. Winstom & Sons, Washington, DC

Richard J, Constantinidis J (1970) Les démences de la vieillesse. Notions acquises et problèmes cliniques actuels. Confrontation Psychiatriques 3:39–61

Schwartz MF (1990) Introduction to chapter 5: Neuropsychology of Alzheimer's disease: the case for subgroups by A Martin. In: Schwartz MJ (ed) Modular deficits in Alzheimer-type dementia. MIT Press, Cambridge, p 143

Ska B, Joanette Y, Poissant A, Béland R, Lecours AR (1990) Language disorders in dementia of the Alzheimer type: Contrastive patterns from a multiple single case study. Abstract of the Academy of Aphasia, 28th Annual Meeting, Baltimore (USA), October 21–23

Valdois S, Joanette Y, Poissant A, Ska B, Dehaut F (1990) Heterogeneity in the cognitive profile of normal elderly. J Clin Exp Neuropsychol 12:4:587–596

Primary Progressive Aphasia:
Sharpening the Focus on a Clinical Syndrome

M.-M. Mesulam and *S. Weintraub*

"Dementia" is a generic term that refers to all conditions which cause the gradual dissolution of cognition, comportment and daily living activities. Not all mental functions are equally affected in individual patients, especially during the first several years of the disease process. The relative degrees of sparing and involvement across specific domains such as attention, memory, language, and comportment lead to the establishment of neuropsychological profiles in dementing diseases.

The single most common neuropsychological profile in adult-onset dementia is characterized by a progressive amnesia. Included in this category are patients who display the insidious appearance and progressive exacerbation of primary memory deficits within the first two years of clinically identifiable onset. Deficits in other domains may coexist and may even be more salient at certain stages of the disease. When caused by degenerative brain diseases (that is when stroke, hydrocephalus, tumor, metabolic factors, etc., are eliminated as etiologies), this neuropsychological profile is identical to the McKhann et al. (1984) criteria for probable Alzheimer's disease (PRAD). In a sample of the first 39 consecutive cases from the Beth Israel-Massachusetts Alzheimer's Disease Research Center (BI-ADRC) that came to autopsy or brain biopsy with a clinical diagnosis of dementia, this profile occurred 21 times and was associated with the multifocal neurofibrillary tangles and neuritic plaques of Alzheimer's disease (AD) in 20 cases (Price et al., in preparation). Experience from other centers yields a concordance of 68–100% between the clinical syndrome of PRAD and the pathological diagnosis of AD (Morris et al., 1988; Risse et al., 1990). Other and less frequent pathological conditions associated with PRAD include nonspecific degenerations, Pick's disease and Lewy body encephalitis (Risse et al., 1990).

Additional neuropsychological profiles associated with dementia include those of progressive comportmental dysfunction and progressive visuospatial disturbances. In six consecutive autopsies of patients with progressive comportmental dysfunction seen in the BIH-ADRC Clinic, the neuropathological examination revealed neuronal loss, gliosis and atrophy predominantly of the frontal lobes. The profile of progressive visuospatial disturbance is associated with a more heterogeneous set of pathophysiological correlates that includes AD, Jakob-Creutzfeldt disease, and probably also nonspecific gliosis and neuronal loss with an emphasis on the parieto-temporo-occipital regions of the brain (see Weintraub and Mesulam, 1993, for review).

F. Boller et al. (Eds.)
Heterogeneity of Alzheimer's Disease
© Springer-Verlag Berlin Heidelberg 1992

Table 1. Clinical definitions

PRAD[a]	PPA[a]
progressive worsening of memory and other cognitive functions	progressive worsening of language (not just speech)
deficits in two ore more areas of cognition	absence of deficits in other domains during the first 2 years or longer
no disturbance of consciousness	no disturbance of consciousness
presence of "dementia" syndrome	no additional signs of a more generalized "dementia"[b] syndrome
absence of systemic disorders or other brain disease that in and of themselves could account for the progressive deficits in memory and other cognitive functions	absence of systemic disorders or other brain disease that in and of themselves could account for the progressive deficits in language

[a] Abbreviations: PRAD, probable Alzheimer's disease, according to the McKhann et al. – NINCDS (1984) criteria; PPA, primary progressive aphasia.
[b] Depending on the definition that one chooses to use, the presence of the progressive aphasic disturbance itself would lead to the classification of these patients as having a dementing syndrome.

This chapter deals with a fourth neuropsychological profile, one that we have identified as primary progressive aphasia (PPA). According to our current definition (Table 1), this diagnosis is made when a gradual dissolution of language (not just speech) is the only salient finding for at least two years and when this deficit becomes the only factor that compromises daily living activities. Attention, memory, visuospatial skills and comportment must be relatively intact during the first two years of the disease. Other deficits of relatively lesser intensity are acceptable if they occur on tasks mediated by the left hemisphere language network (such as word fluency, verbal retrieval, digit span, calculations, ideometor apraxia), if they are secondary to the language defect (due to an inability to process the linguistic or execute the praxis components of the task) and if they are reactive (such as depression and frustration caused by an awareness of the deficits). After the initial two years, deficits in other domains may emerge but the aphasia remains as the most salient feature.

The diagnosis of PPA should not be applied to patients who also develop memory or comportmental disturbances during the first two years of an otherwise progressive aphasia. Neuropsychological testing helps to differentiate PPA from PRAD since a disturbance of memory rules out PPA while it is a necessary criterion for the diagnosis of PRAD (Table 1).

Clinical and Neurodiagnostic Features of Patients with Primary Progressive Aphasia – A Review of the Literature

The existence of slowly progressive language deficits in the context of degenerative disease has been appreciated for nearly 100 years. The reports of Pick

(1892, 1904), Dejerine and Sérieux (1897), Franceschi (1908) and Rosenfeld (1909) provide examples of such patients. Among these cases, Dejerine and Sérieux's (1897) patient and Rosenfeld's (1909) first patient fit our definition of PPA. Dejerine and Sérieux described a patient who developed a state of pure word deafness at the age of 47. Gradual worsening of the language deficit occurred in the absence of other signs of dementia. Within five years, the patient's deficit advanced to a state of Wernicke's aphasia. She died eight years after the emergence of the first symptoms. Autopsy revealed massive bitemporal atrophy with a loss of intracortical fibers and pyramidal cells. The first patient in Rosenfeld's 1909 report (as reviewed by Luzzatti and Poeck, 1991) sought medical advice at the age of 62 with a history of progressive word finding difficulties. Other aspects of cognition and comportment remained relatively intact but some memory disturbances might have been detected at a time when he was examined three years after onset. At autopsy, atrophy and neuronal loss, especially marked in the left temporal lobe, were reported. There is insufficient clinical information to decide if Patient 2 in Pick's 1904 report fits the definition of PPA but the patient reported by Pick in 1892, patients 1 and 3 in his 1904 paper, and the patient reported by Franceschi in 1908 clearly displayed additional and major abnormalities of memory and/or comportment at the very initial stages of gradually progressive aphasic disturbances.

One of the earliest contributions to the modern literature on progressive aphasia was Wechsler's 1977 report of a 60-year-old man with a progressive decline of language function who turned out to have Pick's disease at autopsy (Weschler et al., 1982). As indicated in the 1977 paper, the patient had considerable comportmental disturbances in the early phases of the disease. One year after putative onset, the patient started to shy away from people and became irritable and suspicious. He would catch flies, proceed to pull off their wings and set them afire with matches. Presumably such behavior was not consistent with the patient's previous personality. In view of the early emergence of comportmental disturbances, Wechsler's patient does not fit our current definition of PPA and shares many features with the patients of Pick and Franchesi, where progressive language deficits were associated early in the course of the disease with other comportmental and cognitive difficulties.

In 1982, we described six patients with PPA (Mesulam, 1982). Table 2 lists 63 cases reported during the 10-year period from 1982 to 1992 that fulfill the diagnostic criteria for PPA. Omitted from this list were patients who had deficits other than aphasia in the first two years (such as those in reports by Kobayashi et al., 1990; and Snowden et al., 1989) as well as reports that did not contain enough information to ascertain that the criteria in Table 1 had been fulfilled. In some of the papers reviewed, only some of the patients were included while others were excluded. Some patients have been reported in more than one publication but were entered only once in Table 2. None of the three patients who developed a progressive aphasia in association with Jakob-Creutzfeldt disease was included since the course was too rapid, leading to death within two years after onset (Shuttleworth et al., 1985; Yamanouchi et al., 1986; Mandell et al., 1989).

Table 2. Characteristics of primary progressive aphasia cases in the literature[a]

N	Author, year, Patient		Gender and GNDR onset age[b]	APHS only[c]	focal tests[d]	Focal signs[e]	Aphasia type[f]	Pathology
1	Mesulam, 1982	pt 1	F69	5	+	+	fluent(−)	
2		pt 2	M57	11	+		fluent(−)	
3		pt 3	F48	8	+		nonfluent	FAtr-Bx[g]
4		pt 4	F17	10	+		fluent	
5		pt 5	M54	9	+		fluent	
6		pt 6	M61	6	+		fluent(−)	
7	Heath et al., 1983		F69	4			nonfluent	
8	Assal et al., 1984		F60	4			mixed	
9	Pogacar and Williams, 1984		M56	2	+	+	fluent	AD L > R[h]
10	Kirshner et al., 1984[i]	pt 1	F64	4			fluent	
11		pt 2	M61	10	+		mixed	FAtr-L > R
12		pt 4	M58	4			fluent	FAtr L > R
13	Holland et al., 1985		M66	11			nonfluent	Pick L > R
14	Chawluck et al., 1986	pt 1	F51	4	+		fluent	
15	Case Records, 1986		F68	5			nonfluent	FAtr L > R[j]

Table 2. Continued

N	Author, year, Patient		Gender and GNDR onset age[b]	APHS only[c]	focal tests[d]	Focal signs[e]	Aphasia type[f]	Pathology
16	Hamanaka and Yamagishi, 1986	pt 1	F55	4	+		fluent	
17		pt 2	F60	4	+		mixed	
18	Mehler et al., 1987	pt 1	M54	3	+		nonfluent	FAtr L > R
19	Mehler et al., 1987	pt 2	M53	4	+		nonfluent	
20	Basso et al., 1988		M68	6	+		fluent	
21	Poeck and Luzzatti, 1988	pt 1	F63	3	+		fluent	
22		pt 2	M53	4	+		fluent	
23		pt 3	M45	5	+		fluent	
24	Goulding et al., 1989		M63	3	+	+	nonfluent	
25	De Oliveira et al., 1989		M63	7	+		?mixed	
26	Kushner, 1989		M71	4	+		fluent	
27	Yamamoto et al., 1989	pt 2	F67	6	+		nonfluent	
28	Sapin et al., 1989	pt 1	M66	3	+		fluent	
29		pt 2	M67	2	+		fluent	

Table 2. Continued

N	Author, year, Patient	Gender and GNDR onset age[b]	APHS only[c]	focal tests[d]	Focal signs[e]	Aphasia type[f]	Pathology
30	Graff-Radford et al., 1990	M56	5	+		fluent	Pick
31	Berger and Porch, 1990	F57	5			nonfluent	
32	Green et al., 1990 pt 1	M60	5		+	fluent	
33	pt 2	M60	5			fluent	
34	pt 3	M75	2		+	fluent	
35	pt 4	M57	3		+	nonfluent	FAtr L > R
36	pt 5	F50	2		+	fluent	
37	pt 6	F73	5			fluent	
38	pt 7	M50	3	+		fluent	
39	pt 8	F71	3		+	nonfluent	AD L > R
40	Northen et a., 1990	M63	5	+	+	nonfluent	
41	Scheltens et al. 1990	M54	9	+		fluent	
42	Weintraub et al., 1990 pt 1	M47	9	+		nonfluent	
43	pt 2	M56	6			nonfluent	
44	pt 3	F40	8			nonfluent	

Table 2. Continued

N	Author, year, Patient		Gender and GNDR onset age[b]	APHS only[c]	focal tests[d]	Focal signs[e]	Aphasia type[f]	Pathology
45		pt 4	M74	9			nonfluent	
46	Kempler et al., 1990	pt 3	M58	5	+		fluent	AD
47	Tyrrell et al., 1990	pt 1	M40	4	+		fluent	
48		pt 2	M59	4	+		fluent	
49		pt 5	M54	2	+		fluent	
50		pt 6	M60	2			nonfluent	
51	Delecluse et al., 1990		F66	3	+		nonfluent	
52	Kartsounis et al., 1991		M58	8	+		nonfluent	
53	Tyrrell et al., 1991	pt 2	M59	6			nonfluent	
54	Mendez and Zander, 1991	pt 6	F55	14		+	fluent	
55		pt 9	M61	2	+		nonfluent	
56		pt 12	F59	4	+		nonfluent	
57	Benson and Zaisas, 1991		M58	7	+		fluent	AD
58	McDaniel et al., 1991	pt 1	F62	2	+		nonfluent	

Table 2. Continued

N	Author, year, Patient		Gender and GNDR onset age[b]	APHS only[c]	focal tests[d]	Focal signs[e]	Aphasia type[f]	Pathology
59		pt 2	F73	2	+		mixed	
60	Lippa et al., 1991		M66	3			nonfluent	FAtr L > R[k]
61	Snowden et al., 1992	pt 1	F65	10			nonfluent	
62		pt 4	M63	8	+	+	nonfluent	FAtr L > R
63		pt 5	M59	3	+		nonfluent	

[a] Includes articles published up to February 1992 that we have been able to identify and for which were abstracts in English, French, German, Spanish or Italien. Abbreviations: APHS, aphasia: FAtr, focal atrophy; pt, patient.

[b] Age of onset was determined by history.

[c] Number of years during which the patient experienced a purely aphasic disorder without deficits in other domains.

[d] Neurodiagnostic tests such as EEG, CT, MRI, SPECT and PET were taken into consideration. A plus sign indicates that at least one of these tests showed a selective abnormality of the left hemisphere. A blank indicates that there were either no asymmetries noted or that the relevant tests were not reported.

[e] A plus sign indicates an abnormality of elementary neural function, such as hyperreflexia or facial flattening, on the right side of the body. A blank indicates either the absence of such a finding or the failure to report the elementary neurological examination.

[f] The classification is based on the observations described in the cited report. We placed the most emphasis on the nature of the aphasia at a time when the disease was clearly established rather than at disease onset. Patients with a logopenic anomic aphasia are indicated by the designation of fluent (−).

[g] The information for this patient is based on a biopsy from the left temporal lobe.

[h] The designation of "L > R" indicates that the pathological changes were described as being more severe in the left hemisphere.

[i] Patient numbers refer to those of Kirschner et al., 1984, but the related pathological information is based on Kirshner et al., 1987.

[j] The diagnosis of Pick's disease was proposed in this case but no Pick bodies were detected.

[k] Neuronal achromasia was also reported in this case.

The cases listed in Table 2 demonstrate that the syndrome of PPA can emerge among speakers of Dutch, English, French, German, Italian, Japanese and Portugese. Patient 4 in our 1982 report was a native speaker of Urdu and we have correspondence indicating that PPA has been noted in speakers of Hebrew and Turkish. If one eliminates as an outlier patient 4 of our 1982 series, who developed progressive pure world deafness at the age of 17, the age of onset ranges from 40–75 with a mean of 60 $\pm$ 8 years. The age of onset was below 65 years in 46 patients and at 65 or above in 17 patients. The list in Table 2 contains 40 male and 23 female patients with a diagnosis of PPA.

Determining the type of language disturbance from published records offered a major challenge. In keeping with a common classification system, we designated the aphasias as fluent or nonfluent. Nonfluent aphasias are characterized by agrammatic spontaneous utterances with a reduced phrase length (under four words) and include Broca's aphasia and transcortical motor aphasia. The fluent aphasias include the anomic, conduction, Wernicke and transcortical sensory subtypes (Benson and Geschwind, 1985). If the clinical report of a given patient with PPA described a nonfluent aphasia and also deficits in language comprehension, we defined that patient as having a mixed (global) aphasia. Patients with speech disturbance (i.e., dysarthria) but without definitive proof for additional language difficulties were not included in Table 2. In some patients on whom we had reported in 1982, speech was fluent, in the sense that phrase length was greater than four words and output was syntactically complete, but there were also lengthy word finding pauses, so that the overall rate of language production was decreased. We identified these patients as diplaying a "logopenic" fluent aphasia to emphasize the preservation of grammar and phrase length. These patients are indicated in Table 2 with the designation of fluent(–). According to these criteria, Table 2 contains 31 patients with fluent aphasias, 28 with nonfluent aphasias, and 5 patients with a mixed aphasia.

Time of onset was also difficult to pinpoint and, in most reports, was based on unstructured interviews with the patient or family members. The time of onset for additional deficits in other domains of cognition and comportment was inferred by historical information and neuropsychological test results. Based on this type of information, we estimated the interval during which the patients with PPA had a "pure" aphasia without other significant cognitive or comportmental deficits (except for dyscalculia, apraxia and reactive dystymia). Table 2 shows that the mean duration of this interval was 5.2 $\pm$ 2.8 years and that there were six patients who displayed a relatively isolated progressive aphasia for 10 years or longer. It is important to realize that these numbers underestimate the duration of the isolated aphasia, since additional cognitive or comportmental deficits had not yet emerged at the time of the last examination of some patients and since some of the observed non-verbal deficits might have been secondary to the processing difficulties imposed by the severe aphasia.

Focal neurological signs, such as right-sided weakness, right facial flattening, right-sided hyperreflexia, right body posturing, right upper extremity tremor or a right-sided Babinski sign, were reported in 11 (17%) of the patients. Asymmetrical neurodiagnostic abnormalities over the left fronto-perisylvian region were reported in 41 (65%) of the patients. The most frequent findings were computerized tomographic (CT) or magnetic resonance (MR) scans, with asymmetrically widened sylvian fissures and frontal horns on the left, and electroencephalograms (EEG), demonstrating asymmetrical slowing on the left and reduced oxygen or glucose metabolisms and blood flow as determined by positron emission tomography (PET) or single photon emission computerized tomography (SPECT) in the left frontal-perisylvian regions. In some patients, the reduced metabolic activity determined by PET was confined to the left hemisphere, whereas in others there were also lesser abnormalities in the right hemisphere (Chawluck et al., 1986; Tyrell et al., 1990). The focality of the atrophy and the associated lucencies seen on CT scans occasionally raised the possibility of strokes. However, angiography or noninvasive diagnostic evaluation of the cerebral vasculature was invariably negative, patients rarely had risk factors for stroke and CT and MR scans in several reports provided evidence for a progressive atrophy over time.

A Clinical and Neuropsychological Picture of Patients with Primary Progressive Aphasia – Our Experience

On initial clinical encounter, the patient with PPA looks much more like a patient with focal stroke than one with dementia. The patient tends to be alert, attentive, cooperative, concerned with the predicament, aware of the deficit and remarkably adept at communicating despite the aphasia, by writing when nearly mute or by pantomime and gesture when necessary.

The patient is almost always the first to detect the presence of the language problem in the form of increased effort (or slowing) during word-finding and decreased efficiency in coming up with the most appropriate of several equally acceptable but perhaps not equally effective words. For several years, the patient may be the only one to notice the difficulty. One of our patients, who later became mute in the context of PPA, was sent to a psychiatrist in the early years of her condition to investigate the possibility of hypochondriasis.

Except for rare cases in which the difficulty may emerge in the form of word deafness (i.e., the patient of Dejerine and Sérieux and also patient 4 in our 1982 report), initial objective evidence for the language difficulty is almost always demonstrated on tests of naming. The naming deficit usually leads to long word-finding pauses that give spontaneous speech a logopenic quality. The naming difficulty characteristically leads to phonemic rather than semantic paraphasias (Weintraub et al., 1990). The earliest difficulties may be detected in the naming of geometric forms and body parts at the same time that other classes of objects are named correctly. In the initial stages, the patients is usually able to point to the correct object when the word is provided by the examiner despite being unable to name it spontaneously. This "one-way" naming deficit indicates the preservation of word "recognition" at a time when there is an impairment of word "retrieval".

Some patients remain at this stage of an anomic aphasia whereas others progress to develop more severe fluent or nonfluent aphasias. In the most advanced cases, mixed (global) aphasias can emerge. Writing and reading can show an relative sparing and the patient may bring a writing pad in an attempt to communicate with the examiner. The patients with the anomic and non-fluent aphasias are the easiest to diagnose as having PPA since the preserved comprehension enables them to give the clearest indication of intact performance in other domains. However, patients with nonfluent aphasias may also have severe ideomotor apraxia and may consequently say or signal "no" when they mean "yes," making conventional testing difficult to interpret. One patient would push the accelerator pedal when she meant to use the left foot for the clutch and had to stop driving because of the apraxia rather than because of other cognitive limitations.

In patients with the nonfluent aphasias (i.e., Broca's aphasia or transcortical motor aphasia), phrase length is diminished, naming is poor, there is almost always dysarthria and the output (spoken or written) tends to be terse but effective in communicating intent. Repetition is decreased in Broca's aphasia but is preserved in transcortical motor aphasia. Writing is never completely spared but can be better than spoken language, so that a patient may be able to write the name of an object that he is unable to utter. In some patients who may have extremely labored and dysarthric spontaneous speech output, singing may improve speech intelligibility. The patients with the nonfluent aphasias also demonstrate a characteristic agrammatism. Their spoken and written language tends to show a paucity of grammatical relational words and morphological markers. While these patients may have excellent comprehension for most conversation, they start to show difficulties with syntactically difficult constructions such as those that include passive voice and embedded clauses. When asked to repeat, they have a greater difficulty with small grammatical words (prepositions, pronouns, etc.) than with semantically rich substantives. This discrepancy is also apparent when reading. For example, a patient may be much faster at detecting the written form of the word "hippopotamus" than the word "it" in a list of 10 words. Buccofacial apraxia is common, especially for pharyngeal movements, constructions may show minor difficulties and calculations are impaired. These additional difficulties are also seen in patients who develop nonfluent aphasias on the basis of focal strokes in parts of the left hemisphere language network.

Patients with the Wernicke and transcortical sensory subtypes of fluent aphasias are the most difficult to assess because of the associated comprehension difficulties.

Transcortical sensory aphasia is differentiated from Wernicke's aphasia by the preservation of repetition. The comprehension impairment in some of these patients is at the level of sentences whereas in others it is at the level of single words. For example, they can neither retrieve the appropriate word for an object they are shown nor match the word with the appropriate object even at a time when they can accurately describe its use. This conditions is defined as a "two-way" naming deficit.

When comprehension is impaired, the patient may not understand verbal instructions, so that attention, memory and visuospatial skills may be difficult to assess. Some of the patients with the fluent aphasias may also show agitation and lack of concern, but it is important to remember that such comportmental disturbances are also seen in patients who develop Wernicke's aphasia in the context of focal strokes.

The assessment of cognitive and comportmental domains in patients with comprehension deficits is a challenging task that requires considerable improvisation. For example, one patient with a fluent PPA was intitially thought to be disoriented because he could not come up with accurate answers related to temporal orientation and topographic location. When given a calendar, however, the patient quickly pointed to the correct date and when provided with a map he was able to point to his location even though he was being examined in a city far from his home.

The most critical factor in the differentiation of PPA from PRAD is the integrity of memory function. Some patients with PPA perform well in conventional tests of memory such as the Weschler Memory Scale, the Rey-Osterrieth Complex Figure, the Rey Auditory Verbal Learning List, and the Three Words Three Shapes Test (Weintraub et al., 1990). In other patients, however, there may be abnormalities in verbally mediated memory tasks. If scores of non-verbal memory tests are normal and if the daily living activities do not give evidence for abnormal forgetting, we assume that memory function is relatively spared and that the abnormal test scores reflect difficulties that are secondary to the aphasia.

In evaluating areas other than memory, we find the Visual Span subtest of the WMS-R helpful for assessing attention, the Facial Recognition and Judgment of Line Orientation tests for assessing visuospatial abilities, and the Visual-Verbal Test or the Raven Progressive Matrices for assessing executive functions and conceptual abilities (Weintraub and Mesulam, 1985). Throughout the assessment, however, the clinician must be prepared to use intuition and inference and to improvise. Giving an aphasic patient a standard test battery (almost always based on verbal instructions if not on verbal responses) and then scoring it in standard form may lead to the erroneous conclusion that the patient has a more widespread (global) dementia.

The extent to which daily living activites can be preserved is the most characteristic feature of PPA. Many patients continue to drive, keep house, handle finances, and perform remarkably well and with exemplary creativity in tasks that can be done without intact language abilities. One patient helped his son build a log cabin while almost mute and could only explain his achievement by bringing a picture to the clinic and demonstrating the activities related to the construction with pantomime. Another patient extended her knowledge of organic gardening and would use gestures and diagrams to instruct us in the appropriate deployment of nasturtium and marigolds in fending off pests in the organic vegetable patch. One patient who is now mute after four years of PPA carries on with her hobby of solving master-level jigsaw puzzles which adorn her bedroom walls. Two patients learned rudimentary sign language at a time when they were severely aphasic. These anecdotal examples provide clues to the maintenance of non-verbal cognitive skills, motivation and jugdment.

There comes a time, however, when the patient loses all ability to communicate. At that time, it is virtually impossible to make any assessment of mental function except by interpreting gestures, facial expression and demeanor. One patient who is at that state after nine years of PPA continues to attend church and other social functions and to take care of her daily needs, including shopping and paying bills.

A Case Description
(taken from Weintraub et al., 1990, case # 43 on Table 2)

At the age of 56 years, a right-handed banking executive began to experience word-finding difficulty that gradually progressed over the next two years and interfered with his work responsibilities. His wife reported that he was occasionally tearful over his condition but otherwise had no personality changes. Neurologic consultation was sought two years after onset. The computed tomographic scan was normal, as was the electroencephalogram.

The initial elementary neurologic examination did not reveal abnormalities. He was well-dressed, alert, fully oriented, and insightful about his situation. Auditory comprehension was intact. Spontaneous speech was distinctly abnormal with nonfluent output, mild dysarthria, and frequent, predominantly phonemic, paraphasias. Grammatical form was impoverished and limited to simple declaratives and stereotypic utterances. Repetition and oral reading was impaired. Confrontation naming contained frequent phonemic paraphasias. Reading comprehension was only mildly compromised. Spontaneous writing paralleled speech, but sentences to dictation were written relatively well. Apraxia was not present. Performance on virtually all tests of reasoning, memory, and visuospatial skills was within the normal range. He was on medical leave of absence from work because of his communication difficulties, but activities of daily living were otherwise unaffected.

Examination a year later showed relatively little objective change. Because of his communication difficulties, however, the patient had been forced to retire but continued to manage the finances of his family and those of a close friend. Moreover, he expanded his interest in gardening, successfully cultivating species not indigenous to his region.

In the last examination, speech was severely nonfluent, agrammatic, dysarthric, and paraphasic. At times it was unintelligible, but the patient was often able to communicate his needs with rudimentary writing. His oral descriptions of the Cookie Theft picture on initial examination (two years after onset) and the four years later (six years after onset) are shown in Figure 1. Writing both spontaneously and to dictation declined in parallel to spontaneous speech. Deterioration was also noted in repetition, praxis, and confrontation naming. Comprehension was impaired only for complex grammatical constructions. Reading comprehension was mildly impaired.

Memory, reasoning, and visuospatial test scores were relatively stable over time and, by the final examination, some test scores were higher than they had been in the initial examination (Fig. 2). Results from an elementary neurologic examination remained unchanged, with the exception of bilateral dystonic posturing of the upper limbs on complex gait. Insight, judgment, and comport-

2 Years Post Onset:

"Ah....the kids in the cookie jar. The boy is
falling over. The sink is stopped up. Water
flowning on the ....fall on the floor. It's summer
time. The window is open. She's washing dishes and
drying dishes.

6 Years Post Onset:

"The washin..fell...the. laid...wash...oh....chamney
..chimney..(wrote "china)* The spickin...goin..slipping...
off...on the floor. the...bee...(wrote "boy)* The
bee...seep...slip...slip..chair. Girl is..cookies."

* Due to severe dysarthria, the patient was permitted to
write words that were unintelligible.

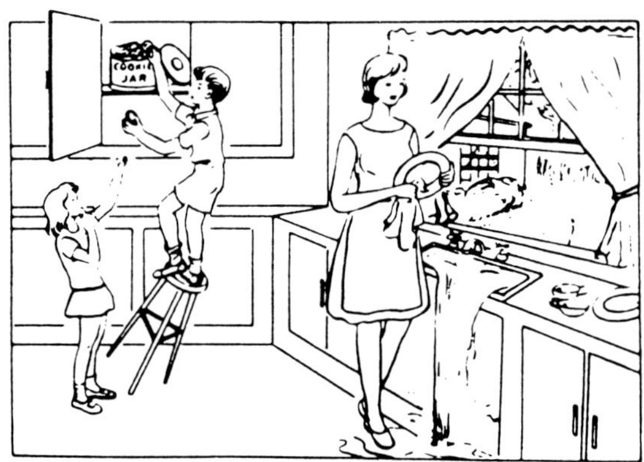

Fig. 1. Oral descriptions of the Cookie Theft picture from the Boston Diagnostic Aphasia Examination taken two and six years after onset. The deterioration is obvious.

ment were maintained, and he continued to offer sound financial advice to his family and friends. He made use of a communication notebook to enhance participation in conversations.

Nature of the Pathological Lesion

Of the 63 cases listed in Table 2, tissue information has been obtained on only 13, one by biopsy and 12 by autopsy. In four of these patients, a diagnosis of Alzheimer's disease (AD) was reached. In one of these four AD cases, the distribution of plaques and tangles was somewhat unusual, since neurofibrillary tangles were distinctly rare in the nucleus basalis and in neocortical areas (Benson and Zaias, 1991). Furthermore, another patient who is included in Table 2 with a pathological diagnosis of AD, the patient of Pogacar and Williams (1984), appears to have displayed considerable deficits in domains other than language, probably within the initial two years, and therefore consti-

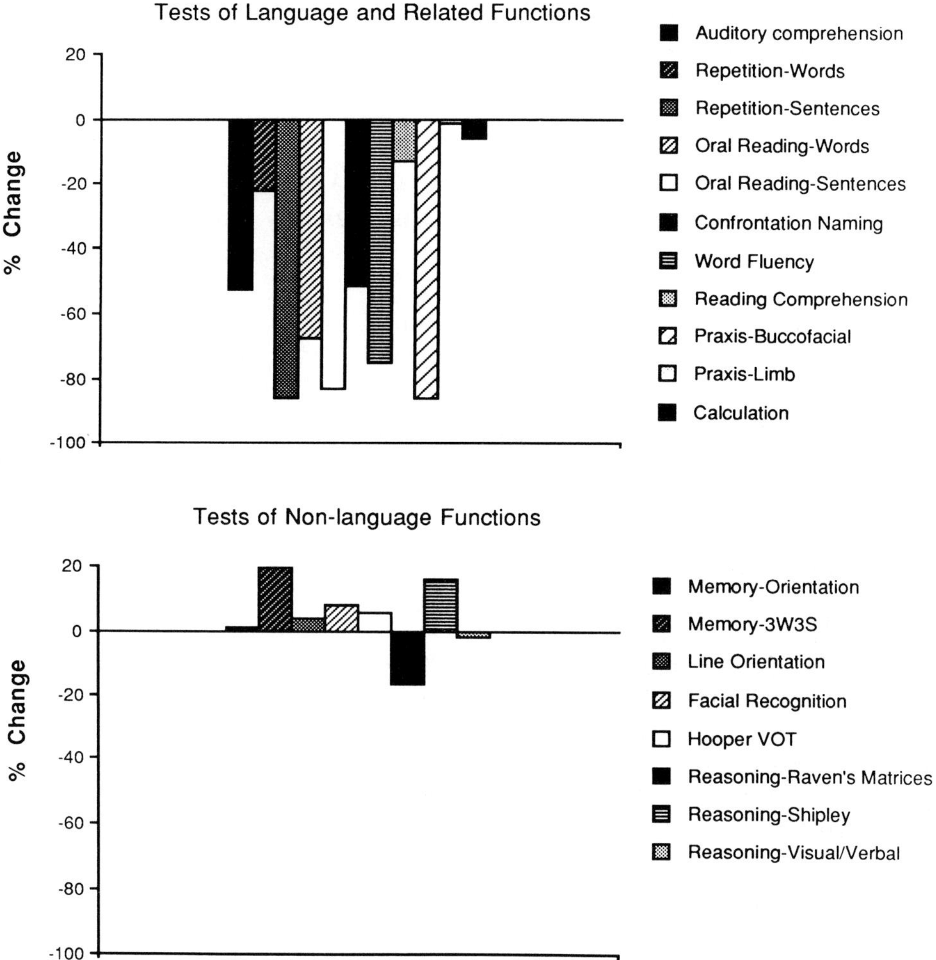

Fig. 2. Percent of change in test scores during a four year interval, from two to six years after onset. 3W3S, Three Words-Three Shapes Test; Hooper VOT, Hooper Visual Organization Test; Raven's Matrices, Raven's Progressive Matrices; Shipley, Shipley-Hartford Institute of Living Scale; and Visual/Verbal, Visual-Verbal Test. Refer to Weintraub et al., 1990 for raw scores.

tutes a borderline example of PPA. In two patients, Pick bodies were identified and a diagnosis of Pick's disease was established (Holland et al., 1985; Graff-Radford et al., 1990). In the remaining seven cases, nonspecific neuronal loss with gliosis and some spongioform changes were reported. In one of these cases, the additional observation of neuronal achromasia was made (Lippa et al., 1991). In virtually all of the cases that came to autopsy, the fronto-perisylvian regions of the left hemisphere were the most affected. In one case where biochemical analyses were undertaken, cortical somatostatin was decreased but cortical choline acetyltransferase was not (Mehler et al., 1987).

The neuropathological experience in the group of patients with PPA is very limited and a considerably different picture may emerge as additional cases come to autopsy.

Primary Progressive Aphasia Compared to Clinically Diagnosed Probable Alzheimer's Disease and Pathologically Proven Alzheimer's Disease

PPA and PRAD represent two non-overlapping clinical syndromes. In Table 3, three groups of patients are compared: the 63 patients in Table 2 make up the PPA group, the first 63 consecutive cases of PRAD in the BI-ADRC core sample of 300 patients make up the PRAD group, and 20 consecutive patients with the pathological diagnosis of AD, where both the clinical and pathological examinations were done in our clinic, make up the AD group.

In the PPA group, disease onset was below the age of 65 (presenile) in 73% of the patients and at the age of 65 or older in 27%. This ratio was reversed for PRAD, where onset below the age of 65 occurred in 32% of the patients and at, or above, the age of 65 in 68%. In the AD group, the age of onset (70% at or above 65 and 30% below the age of 65) was essentially identical to that of PRAD. Of the 63 patients with PPA, 64% were male and 36% female. This ratio was also reversed in the PRAD group, where 21% of the patients were male and 79% were female. In the AD group, 35% of the patients were male and 65% were female, a ratio that was very similar to that of PRAD but very different from that of PPA. To eliminate the possibility that the gender difference was secondary to the difference in age of onset, we also looked at the subset of PRAD cases with onset under the age 65. In that subset of 20 cases, 70% of the patients were female and 30% male, a distribution that remained distinctly different from that seen in the PPA sample. The prevalence of females in PRAD has been described in numerous epidemiological studies (Fratiglioni et al., 1991; Bachman et al., 1992). Since the total sample of PPA is relatively small, however, it is conceivable that there will be changes in the profile of gender and age of onset as additional patients are added to the list in Table 2.

Progressive aphasic disturbances are very common in PRAD and in pathologically confirmed cases of AD. In the BIH-ADRC Clinical Core sample of 20 consecutive cases of AD, 17 had a disturbance of language at initial examination (Price et al., in preparation). In PRAD, the incidence of language difficulties varies from 36% to 100% depending on disease severity (Faber-Langendoen et al., 1988). In both PRAD and AD, the associated language disturbances are almost exclusively of the fluent type, and nonfluent aphasia such as Broca's aphasia or transcortical motor aphasia have not been observed (Appel et al., 1982; Price et al., in preparation). In patients with PPA, however 44% of the aphasias were nonfluent (Broca or transcortical motor) and even some of the aphasias that we classified as fluent were distinguished by a logopenic output.

Table 3. Comparisons of primary progressive aphasia, probable Alzheimer's Disease and Alheimer's Disease

	PPA[a]	PRAD[b]	AD[c]
Onset ≥ 65	27%	68%	70%
Onset < 65	73%	32%	30%
Male	64%	21%	35%
Female	36%	79%	65%
Fluent	48%[d]	100%[e]	100%[f]
Non-fluent	44%	0	0
AD pathology	31%[g]	68–100%[h]	100%
Non-AD pathology	69%	32–0%	0%

[a] The numbers are based on the sample of 63 cases listed in Table 1.

[b] The numbers for age of onset and gender are based on a sample of the first consecutive 63 cases of PRAD entered into our clinical data base.

[c] The numbers are based on a sample of 20 consecutive cases of autopsy confirmed AD cases from our clinic.

[d] Logopenic aphasias are included in the fluent group. The four patients with mixed (global) aphasias were not included in any of the two groups.

[e] This information is based on the report of Appell et al. (1982). Not all PRAD patients had aphasic disturbances. However, those that did had only fluent aphasia subtypes.

[f] Seventeen of the 20 AD cases had language deficits at initial examination. Only fluent aphasias were encountered. None of the patients developed a non-fluent aphasia (Broca or transcortical Motor) at any point in the course of the disease.

[g] The total sample consists of the 13 cases from Table 2 for which there is tissue information.

[h] This range is derived from the reports of Morris et al. (1988) and Risse et al. (1980). In our sample 20 of 21 patients (95%) with clinically defined PRAD who came to autopsy had AD.

These considerations suggest that PPA and PRAD are not only phenomenologically different but that they also represent two different (though perhaps partially overlapping) pools of susceptibilities, both with respect to individuals at risk and regions of the brain that are selectively affected. It also appears that the characteristics of the PRAD group are nearly indistinguishable from those of pathologically confirmed patients with AD, whereas the charactistics of the PPA group are distinctly different from those of the AD group.

In the BI-ADRC sample of 39 consecutive autopsy cases of dementia, 21 patients had the clinical profile of PRAD and 20 of these, or 95%, were associated with the pathological features of AD. In contrast, at most 31% of the PPA patients for whom there is pathological information have an underlying neuropathological process consistent with AD. It should be noted that three of the four PPA patients with AD pathology had a fluent aphasia. If only the PPA patients with nonfluent aphasias are considered (n = 28), only one of seven cases with neuropathological examination (14%) had the findings of AD. These figures show that PPA has more than twice the likelihood of being associated with non-AD pathology than does PRAD (69% versus a maximum of 32%). It also appears that a progressive, nonfluent aphasia is, by itself, a very strong predictor of non-AD pathology.

Is Primary Progressive Aphasia a Disease, a Subtype of Alzheimer's Disease, a Precursor to Dementia? How Heterogeneous is it?

Is PPA a disease? The literature on PPA contains several themes that have fueled considerable discussion. In our initial report of 1982, and on several occasions since then, we stated that PPA is likely to represent a "syndrome" rather than a "disease" (Mesulam, 1982, 1987; Weintraub et al., 1990). A disease, such as AD, is based on at least one dimension of pathophysiological uniformity at the neuropathological or etiological level. A syndrome, on the other hand, is uniform only at the semiological level and may be associated with one of several diseases that collectively constitute the list of its differential diagnoses.

Both PPA and PRAD are syndromes but with substantially different implications for underlying pathophysiology. In PRAD, the incidence of multifocal plaques and tangles is very high – nearly 95–100% according to some authors – whereas in PPA this probability is approximately 30% and becomes even lower if one takes into account only those patients with a nonfluent aphasia.

PPA is neuropathologically heterogeneous in the sense that it can be associated with several entities including focal cortical degeneration, cortical achromasia, Pick's disease and Alzheimer's disease. PRAD is also a heterogeneous syndrome in the sense that it can be associated not only with pathologically proven Alzheimer's disease but also with Pick's disease, nonspecific degeneration and Lewy body encephalitis. However, the probability of finding each of these neuropathological entities varies when PPA is compared to PRAD (Fig. 3).

Is PPA heterogeneous? The syndrome of PPA is clinically heterogeneous as well: some patients can have a fluent aphasia while others have a nonfluent aphasia, and some can show and extremely indolent clinical progression while others deteriorate more rapidly. A far greater degree of heterogeneity is introduced if the definition of PPA indicated in Table 1 is not followed, particularly

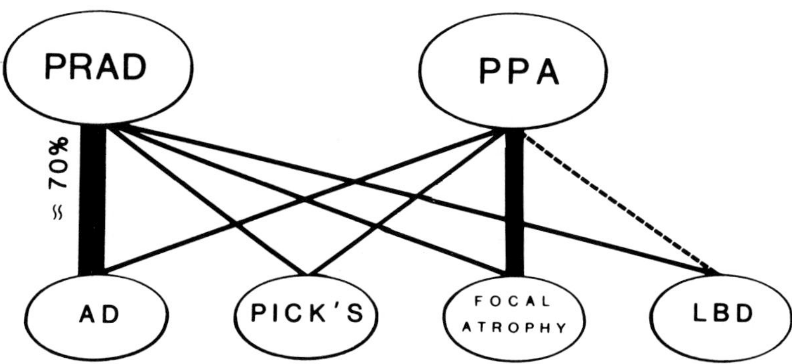

Fig. 3. The relationship between clinical and pathologic planes. Autopsy-verified cases have shown that the clinical diagnosis of probable Alzheimer's disease (PRAD) is associated most frequently with the multifocal plaque-tangle clusters diagnostic of Alzheimer's disease (AD) and less often with Pick's disease (Pick's) and cortical Lewy bodies (LBD). Primary progressive aphasia (PPA), in comparison, is associated most frequently with nonspecific focal atrophy and less often with Pick's disease and Alzheimer's disease.

if PPA becomes equated with all cases of progressive aphasia, including those that have early comportmental and memory deficits. This less restrictive definition encompasses many more patients, many of whom would qualify for the diagnosis of PRAD.

Is PPA a subtype of AD? There are some patients in whom the clinical picture of PPA has been associated with the pathological picture of AD. This probably represents an extremely small proportion of all AD cases, undoubtedly less than 1 in a 100. PPA could therefore join a list that now includes cortical blindness, Balint's syndrome, hemiparesis and right parietal lobe syndrome as one of several rare and idiosyncratic manifestations of AD-like pathology (see, for example, Jagust et al., 1990). It is quite likely that the incidence of AD pathology in PPA will tend to be inflated since some patients will come to autopsy many years after disease onset, in the advanced senium, when the probability of finding neuritic plaques and neurofibrillary tangles is very high even in instances when they may not have been causally related to the emergence of the PPA.

Is PPA a precursor to dementia? Whether PPA is a precursor to dementia is very much dependent on one's definition of dementia. According to the criteria outlined here, PPA could be conceptualized as a dementia confined for at least two years to the domain of language function. The anatomical substrate of language takes the form of a widely distributed network focused around the left perisylvian regions of the human brain (Mesulam, 1990). Individual components of this network also participate in other cognitive domains. It is therefore unlikely that a progressive degenerative disease, even one that is initially confined to the language network, could indefinitely leave other cognitive faculties unscathed. What is truly remarkable is that some patients with PPA experience a relatively isolated language deficit for more than 10 years. This clinical selectivity and the associated anatomical selectivity of the disease for the fronto-perisylvian structures of the left hemisphere reveal a pattern that is very different from that of PRAD, where the selectivity is focused on memory function and the limbic system.

Speculations on the Selective Vulnerability in PPA

Patients with PPA show that a "degenerative" process can selectively (though not necessarily exclusively) target an individual cognitive domain and its corresponding neural network. At least in some patients, the process in PPA may conceivably represent one subset of a larger family of "focal degenerations" which afflict the brain in a regional fashion. When such focal atrophy affects the frontal lobes, the resulting syndrome is identified as progressive comportmental dysfunction. In some patients, the focus of selective involvement is the limbic system and gives rise to a syndrome indistinguishable from PRAD. When the focal atrophy tends to emphasize the left fronto-perisylvian regions, the emergent syndrome is identified as PPA.

The factors that determine the distribution of the selective vulnerability are poorly understood. One of our patients, a retired businessman, had an abscess removed from the temporoparietal region of the left hemisphere when he was 11 years old. Recovery was complete with no residual language deficit. At the age of 70 he experienced the onset of a gradually progressive language deficit. When we examined him six years later, he had a logopenic fluent aphasia but a preservation of function in other domains, a pattern that was consistent with the diagnosis of PPA.

In the course of examining additional patients with suspected PPA, we were also struck by the number of patients reporting a history of early reading or spelling difficulties. We therefore undertook a preliminary study based on nine patients with a clinical diagnosis of PPA and compared them to two control groups, one consisting of 10 patients with a diagnosis of PRAD and a third consisting of 11 nondementing, age-matched control subjects. In a structured interview with subjects and family members, information was obtained about the incidence of developmental learning disabilities in the subjects themselves and in first degree relatives.

Our results show that four of the nine patients with PPA reported an early history of reading and spelling difficulty and two reported difficulty with arithmetic. In contrast, none of the subjects in the other two groups reported early learning difficulties. With respect to relatives, Table 4 shows that a higher incidence of specific learning problems was reported by families of patients with PPA than by families of the other two groups. In one case, there was a family history of dyslexia in several generations. In another, all four siblings reported significant difficulties with writing and spelling and several nieces and nephews were diagnosed as having a learning disability. It is interesting to note that the incidence of PPA is distinctly higher in males, who are also more susceptible to dyslexia and allied learning disabilities.

Table 4. Learning disabilities in probands and first degree relatives[a]

	Learning disability present	Learning disability absent	Probands + relatives
PPA (n = 9)	18	56	9 + 65
PRAD (n = 10)	3	88	10 + 81
CONTROL (n = 11)	2	88	11 + 79

[a] Chi square (df, 2) =32.41, p < 0.001 (2-tail); PPA vs PRAD,
   Fisher Exact Test p < 0.0001; PPA vs CONTROL, p < 0.001

We therefore wonder if PPA reflects, at least in some patients, the tardive expression of a genetic or acquired vulnerability of left hemisphere language networks. In some patients, the vulnerability may be the only determinant and may by itself lead to nonspecific abiotrophic changes. In others this vulnerability can interact with other factors and may provide the site of least resistance for the initial emergence of pathological processes otherwise consistent with AD or Pick's disease.

Conclusions

We have identified a clinical syndrome, PPA, which is distinguishable from other clinical syndromes such as PRAD. The clinical syndrome of PPA is characterized by a relative preservation of memory and language-independent daily living activities in the face of an indolent but relentless progression of aphasia. The literature that we have been able to access contains reports of 63 patients that fit the criteria for PPA. When compared to patients with either PRAD or the pathological diagnosis of AD, the PPA group contains more males, a higher incidence of onset in the presenium and a greater incidence of nonfluent aphasias. The probability of finding AD-like pathology is 68–100% in PRAD but at most 31% in the PPA sample represented in Table 2.

PRAD and PPA are both clinical syndromes of progressive cognitive alterations, but each has a distinctly different set of probabilities for being associated with specific types of neuropathological processes (Fig. 3). Especially at a time when independent biological markers for the underlying disease processes in dementia are not available, the identification of such clinical syndromes is of considerable heuristic value for predicting the possible nature of the underlying pathophysiology and also for counseling patients and caregivers in matters related to management.

Acknowledgments. We want to thank Leah Christie for expert secretarial assistance. Supported in part by an Alzheimer's Disease Research Center Grant AGO-05134 from the National Institute on Aging.

References

Appell J, Kertesz A, Fisman (1982) A study of language functioning in Alzheimer's patients. Brain Language 17:73–91

Assal G, Favre C, Regli F (1984) Aphasia as a first sign of dementia. In: Wertheimer J, Marois M (eds) Senile dementia: outlook for the future. A. Liss, New York, pp 279–282

Bachman DL, Wolf PA, Linn R, Knoefel JE, Cobb J, Belanger A, D'Agostino RB, White LR (1992) Prevalence of dementia and probable senile dementia of the Alzheimer type in the Framingham study. Neurology 42:115–119

Basso A, Capitani E, Laiacona M (1988) Progressive language impairment without dementia: a case with isolated category specific semantic defect. J Neurol Neurosurg Psychiat 51:1201–1207

Benson DF, Geschwind N (1985) Aphasia and related disorders: A Clinical Approach. In: Mesulam M-M (ed) Principles of behavioral neurology. Contemporary Neurology Series, FA Davis, Philadelphia, pp 193–238

Benson DF, Zaias BW (1991) Progressive aphasia: A case with postmortem correlation. Neuropsychiat Neuropsychol Behav Neurol 4:215–223

Berger ML, Porch BE (1990) A longitudinal study of primary progressive aphasia. Neurology (Suppl 1) 40:198

Case Records of the Massachusetts General Hospital: Weekly Clinicopathological Exercises (1986). Vol 314:111–111

Chawluk JB, Mesulam M-M, Hurtig H, Kushner M, Weintraub S, Saykin A, Rubin N, Alavi A, Reivich M (1986) Slowly progressive aphasia without generalized dementia: Studies with positron emission tomography. Ann Neurol 19:68–74

Dejerine J, Sérieux P (1897) Un cas de surdité verbale pure terminée par aphasie sensorielle, suivi d'autopsie. Soc Biol 1074–1077

DeLecluse F, Andersen AR, Waldemar G, Thomsen A-M, Kjaer L, Lassen NA, Postiglione A (1990) Cerebral blood flow in progressive aphasia without dementia. Brain 113:1395–1404

De Oliveira SAV, De O Castro MJM, Bittencourt PRM (1989) Slowly progressive aphasia followed by Alzheimer's dementia. A case report. Arq Neuro-Psiquiat (Sao Paulo) 47:72–75

Faber-Langendoen K, Morris JC, Knesevich JW, La Barge E, Miller JP, Berg L (1988) Aphasia in senile dementia of the Alzheimer type. Ann Neurol 23:365–370

Franceschi F (1908) Gliosi perivascolare in un caso di demenza afasica. Anali Neurolog (Napoli) 26:281–290

Fratiglioni L, Grut M, Forsell Y, Viitanen M, Graftstrom M, Holmen K, Ericsson K, Backman L, Ahlbom A, Winblad B (1991) Prevalence of Alzheimer's disease and other dementias in an elderly urban population: Relationship with age, sex and education. Neurology 41:1886–1892

Goulding PJ, Northen B, Snowden JS, MacDermott N, Neary D (1989) Progressive aphasia with right-sided extrapyramidal signs: another manifestation of localised cerebral atrophy. J Neurol Neurosurg Psychiat 52:128–130

Graff-Radford NR, Damasio AR, Hyman BT, Hart MN, Tranel D, Damasio H, Van Hoesen GW, Rezai K (1990) Progressive aphasia in a patient with Pick's disease: A Neuropsychological, radiologic and anatomic study. Neurology 40:620–626

Green J, Morris JC, Sandson J, McKeel DW, Miller JW (1990) Progressive aphasia: A precursor of global dementia? Neurology 40:423–429

Hamanaka T, Yamagishi H 1986) Slowly progressive aphasia in the praesenium with much later onset of generalized dementia: report of two cases. Proceedings of the Joint Japan-China Stroke Conference, Hirosaka and Tokyo, Japan pp 33–40

Heath PD, Kennedy P, Kapur N (1983) Slowly progressive aphasia without generalized dementia. Ann Neurol 13:687–688

Holland Al, McBurney DH, Moossy J, Reinmuth OM (1985) The dissolution of language in Pick's disease with neurofibrillary tangles: A case study. Brain Language 24:36–58

Jagust WJ, Davies P, Tiller-Borcich JK, Reed BR (1990) Focal Alzheimer's disease. Neurology 40:14–19

Kartsounis LD, Crellin RF, Crewes H, Toone BK (1991) Primary progressive non-fluent aphasia: a case study. Cortex 27:121–129

Kempler D, Metter EJ, Riege WH, Jackson CA, Benson DF, Hanson WR (1990) Slowly progressive aphasia: three cases with language, memory, CT and PET data. J Neurol Neurosurg Psychiat 53:–987–993

Kirshner HS, Tanridag O, Thurman L, Whetsell WO (1987) Progressive aphasia without dementia: two cases with focal spongiform degeneration. Ann Neurol 22:527–532

Kirshner HS, Webb WG, Kelly MP, Wells CE (1984) Language disturbance: An initial symptom of cortical degenerations and dementia. Arch Neurol 41:491–496

Kobayashi K, Kurachi M, Gyoubu T, Fukutani Y, Inao G, Nakamura I, Yamaguchi N (1990) Progressive dysphasic dementia with localized cerebral atrophy: report of an autopsy. Clin Neuropath 9:254–261

Kushner M (1989) MRI and ^{123}I-iodoamphetamine SPECT imaging of a patient with slowly progressing aphasia. Advances in Functional Neuroimaging (Winter) 17–20

Lippa CF, Cohen R, Smith TW, Drachman DA (1991) Primary progressive aphasia with focal neuronal achromasia. Neurology 41:882–886

Luzzatti C, Poeck K (1991) An early description of slowly progressive aphasia. Arch Neurol 48:228–229

Mandell AM, Alexander MP, Carpenter S (1989) Creutzfeldt-Jakob disease presenting as isolated aphasia. Neurology 39:55–58

McDaniel KD, Wagner MT, Greenspan BS (1991) The role of brain single photon emission computed tomography in the diagnosis of primary progressive aphasia. Arch Neurol 48:1257–1260

McKhann G, Drachman D, Folstein M, Kargman R, Price D, Stadlan EM (1984) Clinical diagnosis of Alzheimer's disease: report of the NINCDS-ADRDA Work Group under the auspices of the Department of Health and Human Services Task Force on Alzheimer's Disease. Neurology 34:939–944

Mehler MF (1988) Mixed transcortical aphasia in nonfamilial dysphasic dementia. Cortex 24:545–554

Mehler MF, Horoupian DS, Davies P, Dickson DW (1987) Reduced somatostatin-like immunoreactivity in cerebral cortex in nonfamilial dyphasic dementia. Neurology 37:1448–1453

Mendez MF, Zander BA (1991) Dementia presenting with aphasia: clinical characteristics. J Neurol Neurosurg Psychiat 54:542–545

Mesulam M-M (1982) Slowly progressive aphasia without generalized dementia. Ann Neurol 11:592–598

Mesulam M-M (1987) Primary progressive aphasia: Differentiation from Alzheimer's disease. Ann Neurol 22:533–534

Mesulam M-M (1990) Large scale neurocognitive networks and distributed processing for attention, language and memory. Ann Neurol 28:597–613

Morris JC, McKeel DW, Fulling K, Torack RM, Berg L (1988) Validation of clinical diagnostic criteria for Alzheimer's disease. Arch Neurol 24:17–22

Northern B, Hopcutt B, Griffiths H (1990) Case study: progressive aphasia without generalized dementia. Aphasiology 4:55–65

Pick A (1892) Über die Beziehungen der senilen Hirnatrophie zur Aphasie. Prager Medicinische Wochenschrift 17:165–167

Pick A (1904) Zur Symptomatologie der linksseitigen Schläfenlappenatrophie. Monatschrf Psychiatr Neurol 16:378–388

Poeck K, Luzzatti C (1988) Slowly progressive aphasia in three patients: The problem of accompanying neuropsychological deficit. Brain 111:151–168

Pogacar S, Williams RS (1984) Alzheimers' disease presenting as slowly progressive aphasia. Rhode Island Med J 67:181–185

Risse SC, Raskind MA, Nochlin D, Sumi SM, Lampe TH, Bird TD, Cubberley L, Peskind ER (1990) Neuropathological findings in patients with clinical diagnoses of probable Alzheimer's disease. Am J Psychiatry 147:168–172

Rosenfeld M (1909) Die partielle Großhirnatrophie. J Psychol Neurol 14:115–130

Sapin LR, Anderson FH, Pulaski PD (1989) Progressive aphasia without dementia: Further documentation. Ann Neurol 25:411–413

Scheltens Ph, Hazenberg GJ, Lindeboom J, Valk J, Wolters EC (1990) A case of progressive aphasia without dementia: "temporal" Pick's disease? J Neurol Neurosurg Psychiat 53:79–80

Shuttleworth EC, Yates AJ, Paltan-Ortiz JD (1985) Case report: Creutzfeldt-Jakob disease presenting as progressive aphasia. J Nat Med Assoc 77:649–656

Snowden JS, Goulding PJ, Neary D (1989) Semantic dementia: a form of circumscribed cerebral atrophy. Behav Neurol 2:167–182

Snowdon JS, Neary D, Mann DMA, Goulding PJ, Testa HJ (1992) Progressive language disorder due to lobar atrophy. Ann Neurol 31:174–183

Tyrrell PJ, Warrington EK, Frackowiak RSJ, Rossor MN (1990) Heterogeneity in progressive aphasia due to focal cortical atrophy. Brain 113:1321–1336

Tyrrell PJ, Kartsounis LD, Frackowiak RSJ, Findley LJ, Rossor MN (1991) Progressive loss of speech output and orofacial dyspraxia associated with frontal lobe metabolism. J Neurol Neurosurg Psychiat 54:351–357

Wechsler AF (1977) Presenile dementia presenting as aphasia. J Neurol Neurosurg Psychiat 40:303–305

Wechsler AF, Verity A, Rosenschein S, Fried I, Scheibel AB (1982) Pick's Disease: A clinical, computed tomographic and histologic study with Golgi impregnation observations. Arch Neurol 39:287–290

Weintraub S, Mesulam M-M (1985) Mental state assessment of young and elderly adults in behavioral neurology. In: Mesulam M-M (ed) Principles of behavioral neurology. Contemporary Neurology Series, FA Davis, Philadelphia, pp 71–168.

Weintraub S, Mesulam M-M (1993) Neuropsychological profiles in dementia. Handbook of Neuropsychology, Elsevier

Weintraub S, Rubin NP, Mesulam M-M (1990) Primary progressive aphasia: Longitudinal course, neuropsychological profile and language features. Arch Neurol 47:1329–1335

Yamamoto T, Fukuyama H, Yamadori A (1989) Two cases of slowly progressive aphasia without generalized dementia (Mesulam). A study with CT, MRI and [^{18}F] FDG-PET. Neurol Med (Japan) 31:183–190

Yamanouchi H, Budka H, Vass K (1986) Unilateral Creutzfeldt-Jakob disease. Neurology 36:1517–1520

Therapeutic Drug Trials and Heterogeneity of Alzheimer's Disease

F. Forette, P. Bert, V. Breuil, and *F. Boller*

Alzheimer's disease (AD) varies from one patient to another in terms of age of onset, course, clinical and behavioral features, anatomical and neurochemical lesions, and mode of inheritance (Friedland, 1988). It is not clear whether these variations represent different points of a continuum or true heterogeneity of the disease. A new aspect of possible heterogeneity has been revealed by the recent finding that AD patients differ in their response to pharmacologic interventions. The purpose of this paper is to review specific and non-specific procedures that have been used to evaluate wheter this variability corresponds to actual differences in the disease process.

Non-specific Procedures

A non-specific procedure, the enrichment protocol, was recently tried in some studies involving tetrahydroaminoacridine, known as Tacrine or THA. Thal and his collaborators (1983) were probably the first to suggest that an "enrichment design" (Gracon et al., 1991; Mohr and Chase, 1991) might be useful for investigating cholinesterase inhibitors and other drugs with relatively narrow therapeutic windows. The enrichment design consists in setting up a titration phase to determine the best dose for a given patient, and to exclude patients who are considered non-responders. By selecting patients on the basis of their ability to respond to a given treatment, this design is suitable to an area where one expects heterogeneity. Indeed, the efficacy of a drug is more likely to appear if the double-blind phase of the trial is run on a homogeneous subpopulation of patients on which a measurable benefit has already been shown. As we shall see, however, a number of factors can invalidate the results of the "responders" determination in this designs.

The enrichment design was used in both the American and French studies (Davies and Thal, 1992). The patients included in the study met NINCDS/ADRDA criteria for the diagnosis of probable AD. The patients were mildly to moderately impaired in terms of cognitive and memory deficits as demonstrated by a score of 10 to 26 on the Mini-Mental State Examination (MMS) (Folstein et al., 1975). All patients were 50 years of age or older and were otherwise in good to excellent heath. Patients could not be on concurrent medications with intrinsic CNS activity.

F. Boller et al. (Eds.)
Heterogeneity of Alzheimer's Disease
© Springer-Verlag Berlin Heidelberg 1992

Patients who were found eligible to enter the study were initially randomized to one of three titration sequences and were treated with placebo, 40 mg/day and 80 mg/day of Tacrine for two weecks each during a six-week, double-blind dose-titration phase. During this phase, patients were assessed on the Alzheimer's Disease Assessment Scale (ADAS) following the completion of each two-week treatment period.

The patients then entered a two-week washout period which allowed time for determination of the "best dose." This phase also functioned as the baseline for efficacy and safety assessment. It was initially thought that a two-week washout would be sufficient to allow patients to return to their baseline level of functioning, but in fact, this did not occur and patients were not the same when they entered the parallel double-blind phase due to the carry-over effect of Tacrine.

"Best-dose" was defined as the dose of Tacrine producing at least a four-point reduction (which indicates improvement) on the ADAS total score when compared to the score on the blinded placebo. Longitudinal studies indicate that untreated AD patients show an average four-points increase on this scale over a six-month period.

The French study had a secondary criterion. If the patient did not achieve a best dose using the first critererion, then the dose of Tacrine producing at least a 9-point reduction in ADAS total score compared to the ADAS total score at screening was considered the best dose. This determination also takes into account the patient's ability to tolerate the selected dose.

Patients who did not show a beneficial response or "best dose" were dropped from the study. The patients with a best dose were randomized once again to either their best dose of Tacrine (40 or 80 mg/day) or to placebo and then entered the double-blind parallel phase, which lasted six weeks.

After completing the double-blind phase, patients entered the sustained active phase. Following the completion of the sustained-active phase, patients were given the option to continue with treatment during an open label phase. As a consequece, some French patients now have been on Tacrine for more than 4 years.

The French study was conducted at 19 sites throughout France. A total of 280 patients entered the study. There was a greater percentage of women.The mean age was 69 years. A mean MMS score of 19 at screening indicated that patients were mildly to moderately impaired. Date for 242 patients were evaluable for a best dose. Of these, 140 (54%) achieved a best dose. The majority of patients had a best dose of 80 mg/day of Tacrine. An analysis of the distribution of best doses by titration sequences showed that 61% of patients in sequence Placebo-40–80 achieved a best dose of Tacrine, compared with 54% in sequence 40-Placebo-80 and 45% in sequence 40–80-Placebo.

These results showed that the percentage of best doses was higher when the sequence of treatment started with the placebo period which, therefore, was not "contaminated" by the former administration of the active product. This suggests that best-dose determinations may have been confounded by a carry-over effect in patients who received Tacrine before placebo during this phase.

Table 1. Characteristics of patients at screening. French study

	No Best Dose	Best Dose
Number	116 (47%)	130 (53%)
Age	68.8 (7.2)	67.7 (8.0)
Sex Male	45 (47%)	50 (53%)
Female	71 (47%)	80 (53%)
Weight	61.6 (9.9)	61.9 (11)
Preliminary Tests		
MMSE	18.7 (4.6)	18.6 (4.3)
MIS	0.1 (0.4)	0.1(0.5

The "enrichment" design is certainly one of the original aspects of this Tacrine trial, but, as stated above, a number of factors can invalidate the results of the best dose determination in such designs. They include the existence of a carry-over effect of the drug, inadequate duration of each treatment period and dosage limitation or sensitivity of the efficacy criteria.

The THA study undoubtedly suffered from a carry-over effect, as shown by the variation in percentages of best doses according to the sequences of administration of Placebo, 40 mg and 80 mg of Tacrine, and by the fact that the patients did not return to their screening level of functioning during the placebo phase following their first exposure to the drug. Therefore, the baseline for the best dose period was not a "true" baseline. In addition, the dosage of the drug was most probably too limited, as shown by the Levy study (Eagger et al., 1991), which used doses up to 120 mg. Finally, the efficacy criteria may not have been sufficiently sensitive in all patients owing to the use of the ADAS in this population. The presence of these factors may have decreased the percentage of responders and led to a too conservative evaluation of the efficacy of the drug.

An a posteriori detailed analysis of responders (patients with a best dose) compared to non-responders was made to predict the response to treatment. No clear distinction emerged between responders and non-responders in terms of sex, age, weight, race, MMS level or modified ischemic score (MIS) (Table 1).

Some items have not yet been analyzed, in particular, blood pressure level and orthostatic pressure, regulated partly by central cholinergic and noradrenergic system. Indeed, Pomara et al. (1991) reported that the response of 23 AD outpatients to the cholinesterase inhibitor Velnacrine could be predicted on the basis of pretreatment systolic orthostatic pressure (PSOP) changes from a supine to a sitting position. Venalcrine non-responders demonstrated a greater PSOP fall than did responders (9.2 mm Hg versus 2.7 mm Hg, p < 0.002). The authors hypothesized that there could be a clinical AD subtype witht an underlying sympathetic dysfunction. They further speculated that that particular subtype is unresponsive to cholinesterase inhibitor therapy. Schneider et al. (1991) tried to confirm these findings in the patients they studies as part of the US THA protocol. Of the first 40 patients who fulfilled criteria and completed

Table 2. Subtypology of Alzheimer's disease

- Duration of disease
- Rate of progression
- Age of onset
- Behavioral characteristics
- Motor deficits (extrapyramidal signs, myoclonus)
- Mode of inheritance (familial or sporadic)
- Educational level
- History of depression
- Smoking habits

the dose titration phase, 22 improved their score on the total ADAS by four or more points, and thus were considered responders. In this small sample, responders were significantly older (73.8 versus 67.3 years, p =0.009) and had a greater fall in PSOP (8.4 versus –2.0 mm Hg, p = 0.003). These results are opposite to those demonstrated with Venalcrine and this discrepency remains to be explained; the two products have multiple mechanism of action and the small size of the two samples may account for a "by chance" result.

Other factors should probably be considered according to the subtypology of Alzheimer's disease (Table 2): duration of the disease, rate of progression, mode of inheritance (familial or sporadic), behavioral characteristics, motor deficit (extrapyramidal signs, myoclonus), educational level, history of depression, smoking habits, etc. However, up to now, the non-specific approach has been unable to determine any characteristics which could differentiate responders and non responders and then to identify subtypes.

Specific Procedures

A more specific approach consists in trying to determine the neurochemical substrate of different cognitive impairments. A few studies have linked specific neurochemical substances to different aspects of memory disorders (Wolkowitz et al., 1985). As shown in Table 3, acetylcholine could influence memory consolidation and access to longterm memory; since catecholamines are linked to the modulation of memory storage, selective attention and memory retrieval, effort demanding processes; vasopressin could improve acquisition and recall through improved selective attention, etc.

Going one step further, Albert and collaborators (D'Esposito and Albert, 1991) have attempted to define syndromes with distinctive neuropsychological and neurochemical profiles. In one series of studies (Wolfe et al., 1990), his group tried to define a neuropsychological profile consisting of bradyphrenia, depressed mood and extrapyramidal signs irrespective of the traditional diagnostic categories of Alzheimer's disease, Parkinson's disease and major depressive disorders. In the three groups of patients presenting this syndrome, they found a low cerebrospinal fluid homovanillic acid, confirming their hypothesis that this profile could be linked to dopaminergic deficiency. In another series of

Table 3. Neurochemical substrates of memory

Acetlycholine	memory consolidation long term memory
Catecholamines	selective attention memory retrieval memory storage
Gaba	inhibition of acquisition of episodic memory
Vasopressin	acquisition and recall selective attention
ACTH	selective attention
Serotonin	retrieval from long-term memory

studies, Albert et al. (1988) tested the hypothesis that "selected features of aphasia may reflect disruption of specific neurotransmitters systems." They demonstrated that, for example, the dopaminergic agonist bromocriptine could improve a long standing aphasia characterized by hesitancy and impaired initiation of speech. This approach, which cuts across the traditional diagnostic categories, represents a new way of establishing clinico-pathological correlations.

This specific approach may well represent the wave of the future, especially if it can be used in conjunction with instrumental techniques used as pharmacological probes (e.g., EEG data, P-300 latency modification, glucose metabolism analyzed by PET and cerebral blood flow analyzed by SPECT). Alhainen et al. (1991) suggested that a single dose pharmaco-EEG may predict response to THA. Fourteen AD patients received a seven-week THA treatment. Six patients were regarded as responders and eight as non-responders. AD patients as well as controls had a baseline EEG recording and, on the next day, another recording 90 minutes after an oral single dose of 50 mg THA. The relative change from the baseline in the alpha-theta ratio was the most sensitive discriminator of responders and non-responders. On the other hand, Van Gool et al., (1991) failed to demonstrate an effect of THA on P300 latency in 12 AD patients; the cognitive scores were not affected by treatment.

Tune et al. (1991) investigated the effects of acute intravenous administration of physostigmine on cognitive functioning, cerebral glucose metabolism analyzed by PET and cerebral blood flow analyzed by SPECT in 14 AD patients. Only six patients underwent PET-scanning. Although physostigmine enhanced cerebral blood flow in most patients, only one patient showed significant clinical improvement. This patient, however, showed a very pronounced improvement in glucose metabolism. If this finding is confirmed, this method could serve as a reliable pharmacologic tool to predigt drug effect.

Harrel and co-workers (1990) found biological markers to be effective in predicting response to oral physostigmine. Twenty AD patients were classified as physostigmine responders and non-responders based on "a priori" established criteria. Of these nine patients were found to respond to physostigmine, while 11 were classified as non-responders. When compared to non-responders during baseline conditions, responders were found to have higher concentrations of red blood cell (RBC) choline (Ch) and higher ratios of RBC choline to plasma choline. These data also need confirmation.

Conclusion

Of all the heterogeneous features discussed in this volume, the variability in drug response demonstrated in AD patients may well be the most meaningful and argues in favor of the hypothesis that the disease is heterogeneous in many aspects and particularly in biochemical profile and pathogenesis. The existence of responders and non-responders increases the difficulty of drug evaluation, since their characteristics and identification have not yet been established. So far, non specific methods have been unable to predigt effectiveness. Development of more specific approaches, such as PET scan or SPECT, as well as the continuing search for biological markers must be encouraged.

References

Albert M, Bachman D, Morgan A, Helm-Hestabrooks N (1988) Pharmacotherapy for aphasia. Neurology 38:877–879
Alhainen K, Partanen J, Reinikainen K, Laulumaa V, Soininen H, Airaksinen M, Riekkinen P (1991) Discrimination of tetrahydroaminoacridine responders by a single dose pharmaco-EEG in patients with Alzheimer's disease. Neurosc Lett 127:113–116
D'Esposito M, Albert ML (1991) Pharmacology of memory. Mémoire et vieillissement. Paris, Maloine, pp 247–252
Davies K, Thal L (1992) Tacrine in patients with Alzheimer's disease: A double-blind, placebo-controlled multicenter study. New Eng J Med, in press
Eagger SA, Levy R, Sahakian BJ (1991) Tacrine in Alzheimer's disease. Lancet 337:989–992
Folstein MF, Folstein SE, McHugh PR (1975) "Mini Mental State": a practical method for grading the cognitive state of patients for the clinician. J Psychiat Res 12:189–198
Friedland RP (1988) Alzheimer's disease: clinical and biological heterogeneity. Ann Int Med 109:298–311
Gracon SI, Gamzu ER, Mancini ADJ (1991) Multicenter clinical trials. Design considerations, standardization and implementation. Handbook of Clinical Trials. Lisse, Swets Publishing Service
Harrel LE, Jope RS, Falgout J, Callaway R, Avery C, Spiers M, Leli E, Morere D, Halsey JH (1990) Biological and neuropsychological characterization of Physostigmine responders and non-responders in Alzheimer's disease. J Am Geriat Soc 38:113–122
Mohr E, Chase TN (1991) Treatment strategies in primary degenerative dementias. In: Boller F, Grafman J (eds) Handbook of Neuropsychology, Amsterdam, Elsevier, pp 57–78
Pomara N, Deptula D, Singh R (1991) Changes in blood pressure predict response to HP 029 in Alzheimer disease. Psychopharmacol Bull 27:301–307
Schneider L, Lyness S, Pawluczyk S, Gleason R, Sloane R (1991) Do Blood Pressure and Age Predict Response to Tacrine (THA) in Alzheimer's Disease? A Preliminary Report. Psychopharmacol Bull 27:309–314
Thal L, Fuld PA, Masur MS, Sharpless NS (1983) Oral physostigmine and lecithin improve memory in Alzheimer's disease. Ann Neurol 13:491–496
Tune L, Brandt J, Frost J, Harris G, Mayberg H, Steele C, Burns A, Snapp J, Folstein M, Wagner H, Pearlson G (1991) Physostigmine in Alzheimer's disease. effects on cognitive

functioning, cerebral glucose metabolism analysed by emission position tomography and cerebral blood flow analysed by single photon emission tomography. Acta Psychiat Scand 366 (Supp): 61–65

Van Gool WA, Waardenburg J, Meyjes F, Weinstein C, de Wilde A (1991) The effect of tetrahydroaminacridine (THA) on P300 in Alzheimer's disease. Biol Psychiat 3:953–957

Wolfe N, Katz D, Albert M, Almozlino A, Durso R, Smith M, Volicer L (1990) Neuropsychological profile linked to low dopamine: in Alzheimer's disease, major depression and Parkinson's disease. J Neurol, Neurosurg Psychiat 53:915–917

Wolkowitz OM, Tinklenberg JR, Weingartner H (1985) A psychopharmacological perspective of cognitive functions. II Specific pharmacological agents. Neuropsychology 14:133–156

Pro and Con for Heterogeneity of Alzheimer's Disease: A View from an Epidemiologist

L. Amaducci and *A. Lippi*

The possible heterogeneity of Alzheimer's disease (AD) may be discussed from different methodological points of view and discriminating variables. From an epidemiologic point of view, it is most important to consider etiologic subgroups, such as presenile vs senile, sporadic vs familial. They may be significant in etiologic research since different subtypes may have different risk factors. Failure to separate different subgroups in analytic studies and in clinical trials may lead to spurious negative findings.

Descriptive Epidemiology of Dementia and Alzheimer's Disease

At present, descriptive epidemiology of AD is unable to delineate possible subgroups in this disorder.

The prevalence rate of dementia for people aged 65 and older has been estimated to vary from 4.5% (Hasegawa, 1979) to 18.5% (Nielsen, 1963). All studies conducted to date consistently indicate a steep increase in the prevalence rate with age, despite methodological differences across surveys.

Consistent with the prevalence pattern, the incidence of dementia increasses steeply with age. In a population-based survey carried out in the city of Rochester, Minnesota, Schoenberg et al. (1987) found the incidience rate of dementia to be 0.13% in the 60–69 age group, 0.74% in the 70–79 age class, and 2.17% after the age of 80.

Alzheimer's disease(AD) is the most common dementing condition. Available prevalence rates (cases per 100 population, over 65 years) of AD are estimated to range from 0.6 (Shen et al., 1987) in China to 10.3, in the study by Evans at al. (1989), in East Boston, Massachusetts. This variability in the prevalence rates can be influenced by *different definitions of the disease* under study and different case ascertainment procedures. Some investigators (Sulkava et al., 1985) considered only severe dementia, whereas in other studies, mild dementia was also included (Rocca et al., 1990; Brayne and Calloway, 1989). Akesson(1969), who found very low prevalence rates, adopted very restrictive diagnostic criteria. Constant disorientation to time and place was required to make the diagnosis of AD. *Case ascertainment procedures* also differ in various studies. In a small population, Shen et al. (1987) in Beijing found a low prevalence rate, while a more recent Chinese prevalence survey, carried out in Shanghai in a more representative population sample, yielded a

F. Boller et al. (Eds.)
Heterogeneity of Alzheimer's Disease
© Springer-Verlag Berlin Heidelberg 1992

prevalence rate of 2.03 in a population aged 55 years and older (Zhang et al., 1990). Molsa et al. (1982) in Finland and Akesson (1969) in Sweden collected data only from health and social services and reported lower prevalence rates of dementia. By using the door-to-door approach in a population-based survey conducted on all the inhabitants of a district of Stockholm (Fratiglioni et al. (1991) found higher prevalence rates than in previous surveys. However, a collaborative re-analsyis of 1980–1990 prevalence findings of AD in Europe (Rocca et al., 1991) suggests that, when age and sex are taken into account, there are no significant geographic differences in AD prevalence rates across Europe. Moreover, the prevalence rate increases exponentially with advancing age, ranging respectively, 0.3, 3.1 and 10.8% for the age groups 60–69, 70–79, and 80–89. It is still unclear if the same pattern is present in the most advanced ages. On the whole, women have higher prevalence rates than men in the same age category, as was also reported in Shanghai (Zhang et al., 1990), Copiah County, Mississippi (Schoenberg et al., 1985), and Rochester, Minnesota (Schoenberg et al., 1987).

Consistent with the prevalence pattern, *the incidence rate* for AD raises exponentially with age, and, as summarized by Kay (1991), it appears to triple for each additional 10 years of age beyond 65. The rates are consistently higher in females in all the age groups. In a community-based survey in Finland, Molsa et al. (1982) found that the age-specific annual incidence rates for AD were 0.06 cases per 100 in the age class 45–54, and rose to 11.44 per 1000 in the age group of 85 years and older. The incidience rates were higher in females, except for the 45–54 age group. Using the Israeli National Neurological Disease Register as the source of cases in Israel Treves et al. (1986) confirmed the age effect with 0.01 cases per 1000 in the age class 45–49, and 0.87 per 1000 in subjects aged 60 years and older. Females showed higher incidence rates in this group. Moreover, in this study the age-specific incidence rates were higher in the European-American born citizens than in those who were Afro-Asian born.

No significant variations seem to have occurred in AD prevalence and incidence rates across the years. The prevalence of AD in Lund remained stable between 1957 and 1972 for both sexes (Rorsman et al., 1986); similar findings were more recently observed in Rochester in the five-year period 1975–1980 (Beard et al., 1991). These trends are consistent with those observed for incidence (Rorsman et al., 1986). Moreover the slope of the age-specific prevalence and incidence curves is constant across countries, despite important methodological differences across surveys. This age-specific pattern has nosologic implications for the controversy as to whether presenile and senile AD represent two distinct entities. If the presenile and senile forms were different disorders, distinguished by age of onset, the curve of the age-specific incidence rate should be bimodal; however, population-based studies conducted to date do not confirm such a pattern, but rather show a smooth exponential increase with age, suggesting that age by itself is not an important variable in subcategorizing AD. However, the angle of the curve may indicate that the speed of occurrence of the disease may be different in more advanced ages.

Analytic Epidemiology of Alzheimer's Disease

Analytic epidemiology is concerned with the etiology of a disease. It is aimed at identifying the factors associated with a high risk of disease. Our knowledge of risk factors for AD is based principally upon findings coming from retrospective case-control studies. Much evidence suggests a role of genetic factors in the etiology of AD. Case-control studies have shown a positive association with the following hypothesized risk factors: family history of dementia, Down's, syndrome in relatives, advanced age of the mother at subject's birth, and head trauma.

In the case-control study by Amaducci et al. (1986), the presence of dementia in any first-degree relative yielded an odd ratio equal to 6.5 in comparison with hospital controls and over 2.0 in comparison with population controls, where as the presence of dementia in any sibling yielded an odds ratio equal to 11.0 in comparison with hospital controls and over 5.0 in comparison with population controls. Similar findings were made in other case-control studies (Heyman et al., 1984; Shalat et al., 1987; Broe et al., 1990; Graves et al., 1990a; Hofman et al., 1989). The meta-analysis of case-control studies (van Duijn et al., 1991) shows that the overall relative risk of AD for those with at least one first-degree relative with dementia was 3.5 (C.I. = 2.6–4.6). The relative risk decreases with increasing onset age, and was significantly lower in patients who had one first-degree relative with dementia (RR = 2.6; 95% C.I. = 2.0–3.5), as compared to those who had two or more affected relatives (RR = 7.5; 95% C.I. = 3.3–16.7). This latter trend was observed in early onset patients as well in late onset patients. Moreover, there is a true difference in relative risk for late onset AD between those who have an affected sibling (RR = 4.8) and those who have an affected parent (RR = 2.3), suggesting that familial aggregation of late onset AD may be of multifactorial origin.

As for the association of AD with Down's syndrome, several observations have been reported about the development of dementia in older patients with the disorder. An increased frequency of Down's syndrome among relatives of AD patients, as compared to the general population, was first reported in the comparative study by Heston et al. (1982); Whalley et al. (1982), using a similar study design, failed to confirm this finding. Two case-control studies found a significant association between AD and the presence of Down's syndrome in the family (Heyman et al., 1984; Broe et al., 1990). In other case-control studies, such an association was not observed (Amaducci et al., 1986; Ferini-Strambi et al., 1990).

The meta-analysis data (van Dujin et al., 1991) showed a significant association between AD and family history of Down's syndrome (RR = 2.7; 95% C.I: 1.2–5.7), which was stronger in those with a positive family history of dementia.

Since the risk factor of Down's syndrome rises with increasing maternal age, several researchers investigated late maternal age at the subject's birth as a possible risk factor for AD. Three studies (Whalley et al., 1982; Cohen et al., 1982; Urakami et al., 1989) found a significant difference in the mean age of the mother at the subject's birth in cases in respect to the controls. An Italian case-control study (Amaducci et al., 1986) showed a significant association in the comparison of AD cases to population controls. Although the association was suggestive, it did not reach statistical significance in comparison with hospital controls. The association was not demonstrated in other studies.

The meta-analysis of case-control studies (Rocca et al., 1991) found a consistently increased risk of AD for maternal age of 40 years and older (RR = 1.7; 95% C.I. = 1.0–2.9). The association was more evident for women and sporadic cases, supporting the hypothesis that sporadic AD could be considered a subgroup of the disease that is different from familial cases.

This intriguing finding needs further data to test the hypothesis of an alternative nongenetic mechanism, such as the proposed influence of extreme maternal age over the psychological and cognitive development of the child, which could, therefore be predisposed to AD in later life.

The role of genetic factors in the etiology of AD has also been supported by the results of molecular biology studies. A genetic defect was located on chromosome 21 in some families with early-onset AD (St George-Hyslop et al., 1987). This location was not confirmed in two families of Volga-German origin with early onset AD, or in families with late onset AD (Schellenberg et al., 1988). Recent data suggest that AD, from a genetic point of view, is not a single entity, but might result from genetic defects on chromosome 21 and from other genetic or nongenetic factors (St George-Hyslop et al., 1990).

Among hypothesized environmental risk factors for AD, only the association with head trauma has been observed in several case-control studies (Heyman et al., 1984; Mortimer et al., 1985; Graves et al., 1990b). In some other studies (Amaducci et al., 1986; Shalat et al., 1987; Broe et al., 1990; Chandra et al., 1987) head trauma was more frequent in cases than in controls but the difference failed to reach statistical significance. On the other hand, other studies were not able to find any association between head trauma and AD (Soininen and Heinonen, 1982; Ferinie-Strambi et al., 1990). However, the meta-analysis of 11 case-control studies (Mortimer et al., 1991) showed a pooled RR of 1.82 (95% C.I. = 1.26–2.67). Stratified analyses showed a stronger association in males and in cases without a positive family history of dementia.

Finally, it has been suggested that psychosocial factors,such as education and previous psychiatric disorders, may play a role in etiology and/or in the pathogenesis of dementia and AD.

In the meta-analysis of case-control studies no assocation was found between adverse life events, antidepressant treatment and AD. Such an association, was demonstated, however, between history of depression and late onset AD (Jorm et al., 1991).

As for the role of low education as a risk factor for dementia and AD, an interesting relationship between lower education and higher prevalence rates of dementia has been suggested by some prevalence surveys (Zhang et al., 1990; Bonaiuto et al., 1990; Fratiglioni et al., 1991). In an Italian survey (Bonaiuto et al., 1990), the relationship was more evident for dementia as a syndrome and for vascular dementia whereas the association was less clear with AD. In a Swedish study (Fratiglioni et al., 1991), the higher prevalence of dementia in less-educated people was due essentially to a higher prevalence of alcoholic dementia and unspecified type of dementia. These findings indicate a possible relationship with lower education and dementia, but not with AD. Although prevalence studies cannot be considered etiologically valuable, the observation of these trends deserves further assessment by analytic studies to assay the hypothesis pointed out from a lower "brain reserve" that allows the clinical symptoms of dementia to appear at an earlier date during disease progression (Zhang et al., 1990).

In conclusion, given the heterogeneity of risk factors for AD, the distinction between sporadic, familial, and autosomal form of AD, seems useful. However, all of the studies seem to suggest that the most important risk factor in all AD subtypes is advanced age, suggesting that all the proposed risk factors have to be reanalyzed on the basis of data on the biology of aging. Finally, it must be pointed out that AD was originally described as an independent nosological entity (Kraepelin, 1910), and only recently (Katzman et al., 1978) have AD and senile dementia been considered together. It may simply be that the "heterogeneity" is derived from an artificial "homogeneity," created for not strictly scientific reasons.

References

Akesson O (1969) A population study of senile and arterisclerotic psychoses. Human Hered 19:546–566

Amaducci LA, Fratiglioni L, Rocca WA, Fieschi C, Livrea P, Pedone D, Bracco L, Lippi A, Gandolfo C, Bino G (1986) Risk faktors for clinically diagnosed Alzheimer's disease: a case-control study of an Italian population. Neurology 36:922–931

Beard CM, Kokmen E, Offord K, Kurland LT (1991) Is the prevalence of dementia changing? Neurology 41:1911—1914

Bonaiuto S, Rocca WA, Lippi A, Luciani P, Turtù I, Cavarzeran F, Amaducci L (1990) Impact of education and occupation on the prevalence of Alzheimer's disease (AD) and multi-infarct dementia (MID) in Appignano, Macerata Province, Italy. Neurology 40 (suppl 1):346

Brayne C, Calloway P (1989) An epidemiological study of dementia in a rural population of elderly women. Brit J Psychiat 155:214–219

Broe GA, Henderson AS, Creasey H, McCusker E, Korten AE, Jorm AF, Longley W, Anthony JC (1990) A case-control study of Alzheimer's disease in Australia. Neurology 40:1698–1707

Chandra V, Kokmen E, Schoenberg BS (1987) Head injury with loss of consciousness as a risk factor for Alzheimer's disease using prospectively collected data. Neurolgy 37 (suppl. 1):152

Cohen D, Eisdorfer C, Leverenz J (1982) Alzheimer's disease and maternal age. J Am Geriatr Soc 30:656–659

Evans D, Funkenstein H, Albert M, Scherr P, Cook N, Chown M, Hebert L, Hennekens C, Taylor J (1989) Prevalence of Alzheimer's disease in a community population of older persons. JAMA 262:2551–2556

Ferini-Strambi L, Smirne S, Garancini P, Pinto P, Franceschi M (1990) Clinical and epidemiological aspects of Alzheimer's disease with presenile onset: a case-control study. Neuroepidemiology 9:39–49

Fratiglioni L, Grut M, Forsell Y, Viitanen M, Grafström M, Holmen K, Ericsson K, Bäckman L, Ahlbom A, Winblad B (1991) Prevalence of Alzheimer's disease and other dementias in an elderly urban population: relationship with sex and education. Neurology 41:1886–1892

Graves AB, White E, Koepsell T, Reifler BV, van Belle G, Larson EB, Raskind M (1990a) A case-control study of Alzheimer's disease. Ann Neurol 28:140–148

Graves A, White E, Koepsell T, Reifler B, van Belle G, Larson E, Raskind M (1990b) The association between head trauma and Alzheimer's disease. Am J Epidemiol 131:491–501

Hasegawa K (1979) Aspects of community health care of the elderly. Int J Ment Health 8:36–49

Heston LL, Mastri AR, Anderson VE, White J (1982) Dementia of the Alzheimer type: clinical genetics, natural history, and associated conditions. Arch Gen Psychiat 38:1085–1090

Heyman A, Wilkinson WE, Stafford JA, Helms MJ, Sigmon AH, Weinberg T (1984) Alzheimer's disease: a study of epidemiological aspects Ann Neurol 15:335–341

Hofman A, Schulte W, Tanja TA, van Duijn CM, Haaxma R, Lameris AJ, Otten VM, Saan RJ (1989) History of dementia and Parkinson's disease in 1st-degree relatives of patients with Alzheimer's Disease. Neurology 39:1589–1592

Kay D (1991) The epidemiology of dementia: a review of recent work. Rev Clin Gerontol 1:55–66

Katzman R, Terry RD, Bick KL (1978) Alzheimer's disease: senile dementia and related disorders. Aging, Vol 7. Raven Press, New York

Kraepelin E (1910) Psychiatrie: Ein Lehrbuch für Studierende und Artze, von Johann Ambrosius Barthm Leipzig 533–554; 593–632

Jorm AF, van Duijn CM, Chandra V, Fratiglioni L, Graves AB, Heyman A, Kokmen E, Kondo K, Mortimer JA, Rocca WA, Shalat SL, Soininen H, Hofman A (1991) Psychiatric history and related exposures as risk factors for Alzheimer's disease: a collaborative re-analysis of case-control studies. Int J Epidemiol 20 (suppl. 1):S43–S47

Molsa PK, Martilla RJ, Rinne UK (1982) Epidemiology of dementia in a Finnish population. Acta Neurol Scand 65:541–552

Mortimer JA, French LR, Hutton JT, Schuman LM (1985) Head injury as a risk factor for Alzheimer's disease. Neurology 35:264–267

Mortimer JA, van Duijn CM, Chandra V, Fratiglioni L, Graves WA, Shalat SL, Soininen H, Hofman A (1991) Head trauma as a riks factor for Alzheimer's disease: a collaborative re-analysis of case-control studies. Int J Epidemiol 20 (suppl. 1):S28–S35

Nielsen J (1963) Geronto-psychiatric period-prevalence investigation in a geographically delimited population. Acta Psychiatr Scand 38:307–330

Rocca W, Bonaiuto S, Lippi A, Luciani L, Turtù F, Cavarzeran F, Amaducci L (1990) Prevalence of clinically diagnosed Alzheimer's disease and other dementing disorders: A door-to-door survey in Appignano, Macerata Province, Italy. Neurology 40:626–631

Rocca WA, van Duijn CM, Clayton D, Chandra V, Fratiglioni L, Graves AB, Heymen A, Jorm AC, Kokmen E, Kondo K, Mortimer JA, Shalat SL, Soininen H, Hofman A (1991) Maternal age and Alzheimer's disease: a collaborative re-analysis of case-control studies. Int J Epidemiol 20 (suppl 1):S21–S27

Rocca W, Hofman A, Brayne C, Breteler MMB, Clarke M, Copeland JRM, Dartigues J-F, Engedal K, Hagnell O, Heeren TJ, Jonker C, Lindesay J, Lobo A, Mann AH, Mölsä PK, Morgan K, O'Connor DW, da Silva Droux A, Sulkava R, Kay DWK, Amaducci L for the EURODEM Prevalence Research Group (1991) Frequency and distribution of Alzheimer's disease in Europe: A collaborative study of 1980–1990 prevalence findings. Ann Neurol 30:381–390

Rorsman B, Hagnell O, Lanke J (1986) Prevalence and incidence of senile and multi-infarct dementia in the Lundby Study: A comparison between the time periods 1947–1957 and 1957–1972. Neuropsychobiology 15:122–129

Schellenberg GD, Bird TD, Wijsman EM, Moore DK, Boehnke M, Bryant EM, Lampe TH, Nochlin D, Sumi SM, Deeb SS, Beureuther K, Martin GM (1988) Absence of linkage of Chromosome 21q21 markers of familial Alzheimer's disease. Science 241:1507–1509

Schoenberg B, Anderson D, Haerer A (1985) Severe dementia. Prevalence and clinical features in a biracial US population. Arch Neurol 42:740–743

Schoenberg B, Kokmen E, Okazaki H (1987) Alzheimer's disease and other dementing illnesses in a defined United States population: Incidence rates and clinical features. Ann Neurol 22:724–729

Shalat SL, Seltzer B, Pidcock C, Baker EL (1987) Risk factors for Alzheimer's disease: a case-control study. Neurology 37:1630–1633

Shen Y, Li G, Chen C, Zao Y (1987) An epidemiological survey on age-related dementia in an urban area of Beijing. Presented at the WHO International Workshop on Epidemiology of Mental and Neurological Disorders of the Elderly, Beijing, Nov 16–20, 1987.

Soininen H, Heinonen OP (1982) Clinical and aetiological aspects of senile dementia. Euro Neurol 21:401–410

St George-Hyslop PH, Haines JL, Farrer LA, Polinsky R, Van Broeckhoven C, Goate A, Crapper McLachlan DR, Orr H, Bruni AC, Sorbi S, Rainero I, Foncin JF, Pollen D, Cantu J-M, Tupler R, Voskresenskaya N, Mayeux R, Growdon J, Fried VA, Myers RH, Nee L, Backhovens H, Martin J-J, Rossor M, Owen MJ, Mullan M, Percy ME, Karlinsky K, Rich S, Heston L, Montesi M, Mortilla M, Nacmias N, Gusella JF (1990) Genetic linkage studies suggest that Alzheimer's disease is not a single homogeneous disorder. Nature 347:194–197

St George-Hyslop PH, Tanzi RE, Polinsky RJ, Haines JL, Nee L, Watkins PC, Myers RH, Feldman RG, Pollen D, Drachman D, Growdon J, Bruni A, Foncin J-F, Salmon D, Frommelt P, Amaducci L, Sorbi S, Piacentini S, Stewart GD, Hobbs WJ, Conneally PM, Gusella JF (1987) The genetic defect causing familial Alzheimer's disease maps on chromosome 21. Science 235:885–890

Sulkava R, Wikstrom J, Aromaa A, Raitasalo R, Lehtinen V, Lahtela K, Palo J (1985) Prevalence of severe dementia in Finland. Neurology 35:1025–1029

Treves T, Korczyn A, Zilber N, Kahana E, Leibowitz Y, Alter M, Schoenberg B (1986) Presenile dementia in Israel. Arch Neurol 43:26–29

Urakami K, Adachi Y, Takahashi K (1989) A community-based study of parental age at the birth of patients with dementia of Alzheimer type. Arch Neurol 46:38–39

van Duijn CM, Clayton D, Chandra V, Fratiglioni L, Graves AB, Heyman A, Jorm AF, Kokmen E, Kondo K, Mortimer JA, Rocca WA, Shalat SL, Soininen H, Hofman A (1991) Familial aggregation of Alzheimer's disease and related disorders: a collaborative re-analysis of case-control studies. Int J Epidemiol 20 (suppl 1):S13–S20

Whalley LJ, Carothers AD, Collyer S, De Mey R, Frackiewicz A (1982) A study of familial factors in Alzheimer's disease. Brit J Psychiat 140:249–256

Zhang M, Katzman R, Salmon D, Jin H, Cai G, Wang Z, Qu G, Grant I, Yu E, Levy P, Klauber R, Liu T (1990) The prevalence of dementia and Alzheimer's disease in Shanghai, China: Impact of age, gender and education. Ann Neurol 27:428–437

Heterogeneity in Familial Alzheimer's Disease

M. N. Rossor, A. M. Kennedy, and *S. K. Newman*

Alzheimer's original description in 1907 portrayed a 51-year-old woman who died following a dementing illness and who was found to have senile plaques and neurofibrillary tangles throughout the cerebral cortex. Her clinical features were those of profound memory impairment and language and visuospatial deficits. There was no family history reported.

The initial clinical concept of Alzheimer's disease was that of a rare presenile dementia, although subsequent autopsy studies established that the histological features of presenile Alzheimer's disease and senile dementia of the Alzheimer type were qualitatively identical, regardless of the age of the patient (Blessed et al., 1968). This extension of the usage of the term "Alzheimer's disease" to encompass cases of senile dementia with Alzheimer histopathology drew attention to the size of the health problem, with an estimated 500,000 cases in the UK. Alzheimer's disease remains a clinicopathological concept of dementia with neocortical senile plaques and neurofibrillary tangles. However, the histological features are also seen to a limited extent in apparent normal old age; neuropathological criteria have therefore been developed which take into account the variability of age-related changes. Higher tangle and plaque counts are required in the elderly before the neuropathological diagnosis can be accepted (Khachaturian, 1985). Similarly, clinical criteria have been published for the diagnosis of Alzheimer's disease (McKhann et al., 1984) and three levels of diagnosis – definite, probable and possible – are recognised. "Definite" requires histopathological confirmation; "probable" defines a common presentation of dementia with a prominent memory disorder and a progressive course. The specificty and sensitivity are relatively high, in the order of

Table 1. Heterogeneity in Alzheimer's Disease

Sporadic vs Familial
Early Onset vs Late Onset
Extrapyramidal syndrome
AD + cerebellar and pyramidal features (Aikawa et al. 1985)

Focal onset   – dyphasia (Kirshner et al. 1984)
                 – hemisparesis (Jagust et al. 1990)
                 – Visual disorientation (Cogan 1985)

F. Boller et al. (Eds.)
Heterogeneity of Alzheimer's Disease
© Springer-Verlag Berlin Heidelberg 1992

80%. The probable Alzheimer category has a lower specificity but recognises the heterogeneous nature of the disease with atypical presentations. These include apparent plateaus in the progression, presence of a motor disorder and focal onset (Table 1). The motor disorder itself is variable, ranging from an extrapyramidal syndrome with cogwheeling, rigidity and bradykinesia (Mayeux et al., 1985), which may be associated with Lewy bodies at autopsy (Hansen et al., 1990), to a syndrome of predominantly gegenhalten without obvious extrapyramidal features (Tyrrell et al., 1990). Focal presentations include dysphasia (Kirshner et al., 1984), visual disorientation (Cogan, 1985) and cortical sensory loss with hemiparesis (Jagust et al., 1990). These latter examples of heterogeneity are, however, rare; more readily encountered are the differences between early and late onset and between sporadic and familial Alzheimer's disease.

The familial nature of some cases of Alzheimer's disease was not recognised for some 25 years after Alzheimer's description. The early reports of Schottky (1932) and Meggendorfer (1925) suggested the possibility of an hereditary basis, but it was not until the report of Lowenberg and Waggoner (1934) that autosomal dominant familial Alzheimer's disease (FAD) was clearly recognised. Since then a large number of publications have confirmed the existence of FAD pedigress (Nee et al., 1983; Karlinsky et al., 1991; Bird et al., 1988; 1989; Martin et al., 1991). Some of the pedigrees are very extensive (Nee et al., 1983; Martin et al., 1991), and in all cases the disease is transmitted as an autosomal dominant with apparent full penetrance. Estimates of the prevalence of a family history vary. Initially it was though to be rare, but more detailed epidemiological studies suggest that a family history may be found in 5–50% of cases (Heyman 1983; Heston et al., 1981; Fitch et al., 1988; Mohs et al., 1987; Huff et al., 1988; Farrer et al., 1989). The relative contribution of familial cases to late onset disease is difficult to determine because of the censoring of late onset redigrees by death of family members due to other causes, before they may express the FAD phenotype. It is clear, however, from frequent cases of early onset Alzheimer's disease without any family history and discordance between identical twins (Nee et al., 1987) that a genetic aetiology cannot explain all cases of Alzheimer's disease.

With the realisation that Alzheimer's disease is heterogeneous with both familial and sporadic cases, clinical differences, in addition to the presence of a family history, have been sought between the two groups. Published reports of FAD have focused on young onset cases, often with a mean age of onset in the thirties (Lowenberg and Waggoner, 1934; Martin et al., 1991), forties or fifties (Nee et al., 1983; Karlinksy et al., 1991), but this may only reflect the censoring of pedigrees in late onset disease. Clinical features noted by Lowenberg and Waggoner (1934) included myoclonus and seizures, both of which have been commented on frequently in FAD (Kennedy et al., in preparation), and neuropathologically the occurrence of cerebellar plaques has been suggested to be common in FAD and early onset cases (Pro et al., 1980). However, a distinct FAD phenotype cannot be recognised which serves to distinguish FAD from sporadid cases, other than the presence of a family history.

One of the reasons why a distinct FAD clinical syndrome cannot be recognised is that FAD itself may be heterogeneous. Bird et al. (1989) first drew attention to the variability which may occur clinically. In a study of 24 pedigrees, six groups were recognised. One consisted of the cultural isolate of Volga German ancestry (Bird et al., 1988), one family had tangles and no plaques, one had associated anterior horn cell disease and one had associated white matter changes. Two other groups were distinguished on the mean age of onset, with the early age of onset group having a mean onset at age 42 years. The fact that phenotypic heterogeneity may occur within families with the same genetic defect has long been recognised in other neurological diseases such as Huntington's disease and the GM_2 gangliosidoses. An alternative explanation in FAD is that the phenotypic heterogeneity may reflect underlying genetic and allelic heterogeneity.

Initial linkage studies in FAD concentrated on chromosome 21 because of the known associations of trisomy 21 Down's syndrome with the early development of the histopathological changes of Alzheimer's disease. Linkage to anonymous markers on the long arm of chromosome 21 was demonstrated in 1987 (St George-Hyslop et al., 1987) in a group study of four FAD kindreds, which included the large pedigree reported by Nee et al. (1983). Linkage to chromosome 21 was subsequently confirmed in later studies (Goate et al., 1989; Heston et al., 1991). At the same time that linkage was demonstrated, the amyloid precursor protein (APP) gene was cloned and found to be on the long arm of chromosome 21 (Kang et al., 1987; Goldgaber et al., 1987; Tanzi et al., 1987a). The APP gene was a clear candidate gene for the FAD locus and its localization to the long arm of chromosome 21 supported this view. However, families in which the APP gene was excluded as the FAD locus were soon described (Van Broeckhoven et al., 1987; Tanzi et al., 1987b). Moreover, a large collaborative study of multipoint linkage in a large number of families indicated that FAD is genetically heterogeneous with only the group of young onset families showing linkage to chromosome 21 (St George-Hyslop et al., 1990). The Volga German families had already been shown not to be linked to markers on the proximal long arm of chromosome 21 (Schellenberg et al., 1988), and a study of late onset families had demonstrated linkage to chromosome 19 as opposed to 21 (Pericak-Vance et al., 1991). The realization that FAD could be genetically heterogeneous prevented the pooling of families for genetic linkage studies, considerably hampering research in this area. However, the Alzheimer's Disease Research Group at St. Mary's Hospital, London, studied a single FAD kindred which was sufficiently powerful to demonstrate chromosome 21 linkage within the family and, moreover, the APP gene was not excluded. Direct sequencing of exons 16 and 17 which encode the β/A4 amyloid domain of APP revealed a base change resulting in a valine to isoleucine substitution at APP_{717} which cosegregated with the disease (Goate et al., 1991; see Chapter by Hardy; this volume). The substitution lies just outside the C terminal end of the β/A4 amyloid domain and within the membrane. A point mutation within the extracellular component of the β/A4 domain had previously been described in Hereditary Cerebral Haemorrhage with Amyloidosis – Dutch type (HCHWA-D). In this autosomal dominant disease patients devel-

Table 2. Amyloid Precursor Protein Gene Mutations

	Mutation		Clinical Features	
APP_{693}	Glu → Gln	HCHWA-D	Cortical hemorrhage Dementia	Levy et al. (1990)
APP_{717}	Val → Ile	FAD_1	Onset mid 50s ± motor disturbance	Goate et al. (1991)
APP_{717}	Val → Phe	FAD_2	Onset early 40s	Murrell et al. (1991)
APP_{717}	Val → Gly	FAD_3	Onset late 40s Myoclonus	Chartier-Harlin et al. (1991)

op recurrent cerebral haemorrhage, due to amyloid angiopathy, but without plaques or neurofibrillary tangels. Since the initial report of APP_{717} Val-Ile, two other APP mutations in FAD have been reported at the identical site, resulting in valine to phenylalanine and valine to glycine substitutions (Murrell et al., 1991; Chartier-Harlin et al., 1991; Table 2).

It is clear now that APP_{717} mutations are rare. Approximately 150 families have been screened with largely negative results (Schellenberg et al., 1991; Crawford et al., 1991; Hardy and Rossor, unpublished). No case of sporadic Alzheimer's disease has been reported with an APP mutation. Currently there are studies of eight families with APP_{717} Val-Ile mutation which have been published: four families in Japan, one in the USA, one in Canada and two in the UK (Hardy et al., 1991; St George-Hyslop et al., this volume; Hardy, this volume). At the present time only single kindreds with the APP_{717} valine to phenylalanine and APP_{717} valine to glycine mutations have been reported.

Although the reported APP mutations are rare, they provide an ideal opportunity to relate the different phenotypes in FAD to the underlying mutations. Evidence of genetic heterogeneity is provided by chromosome 21 linked and non-linked families (St George-Hyslop et al., 1990) and late onset chromosome 19 linked families (Pericak-Vance et al., 1991). Chromosome 21 linked families have a younger age at onset (St George-Hyslop et al., 1990), but otherwise there are not distinct differences and it is not known whether there is a single alternative locus, for example, chromosome 19, or multiple loci which might be associated with the FAD phenotype.

Variability within the group of APP mutations can also be seen. The most obvious example of phenotypic heterogeneity reflecting allelic heterogeneity at the APP locus is that of HCHWA-D, in which amyloid angiopathy and parenchymal β/A4 amyloid deposits occur without plaques and neurofibrillary tangles. The mutation at APP_{693} results in a glutamate to glutamine substitution. The clinical presentation is with recurrent cerebral haemorrhage, although there is evidence of additional cognitive impairment (Haan et al., 1991). Affected individuals with the APP_{717} mutations have a mean age at onset in the early fifties for APP_{717} valine to isoleucine and APP valine to gylcine, and an earlier age at onset in the forties for APP_{717} valine to phenylalanine mutation

(Goate et al., 1991; Murrell et al., 1991; Chartier-Harlin et al., 1991). All families show a progressive dementia with early memory impairment as the usual presenting feature. Myoclonus is frequent and, together with seizures, is prominent in the APP_{717} valine to glycine family (Kennedy et al., in preparation). In the three UK families studies witht either APP_{717} Val-Ile or APP_{717} Val-Gly, insight is lost early. Within families the clinical features are similar; for example, a prominent motor disorder in the original UK APP_{717}vValine-isoleucine family. However, between families with the same mutation, there is variability (Mullan et al., 1992). Neuropathologically all APP_{717} cases that have come to autopsy have shown widespread neocortical senile plaques and neurofibrillary tangles with β/A4 immunostaining (Mannet al., 1992; Lantos et al., 1992). In the one autopsied case from the initial UK APP_{717} valine-isoleucine family, cortical Lewy bodies were found, but this finding does not appear to be specific to this mutation (Lantos et al., 1992; Mullan et al., 1992).

Age at onset in FAD is variable but relatively constant within families. A study of ages at onset of thirty FAD kindreds revealed that most variance in age at onset occurred between, rather than within, families (Van Duijn et al., 1990). The age at onset may be relatively specific to the different observed mutations, but even within families variability can be expected (Kennedy et al., in preparation). Variability of onset, rate of progression and age at onset may be relatively specific to a given mutation, but epigenetic factors are likely to have a major influence. FAD kindreds with known mutations provide an ideal opportunity for studying epigenetic factors that might determine the Alzheimer phenotypes. At the present time most cases studies have established dementia, when subtle variations in phenotype may be difficult to observe. We have identified 20 kindred at the Alzheimer's Disease Research Group at St. Mary's Hospital, three of which have identified APP_{717} mutations. Longitudinal follow up includes serial neuropsychological and neurological assessment, MRI and positron emission tomography (PET). Mode of presentation appears relatively constant within families, and the epigenetic factors which might influence age at onset and progression are being sought.

References

Aikwawa H, Suziki K, Iwasaki Y, Iizuka R (1985) Atypical Alzheimer's disease with spastic paresis and ataxia. Ann Neurol 17:297–300

Bird T, Lampe T, Nemens E, Miner G, Sumi S, Schellenberg G (1988) Familial Alzheimer's Disease in American descendants of the Volga Germans: probable genetic founder effect. Ann Neurol 23:25–31

Bird TD, Sumi SD, Nemens EJ (1989) Phenotypic heterogeneity in Familial Alzheimer's disease: a study of 24 kindreds. Ann Neurol 25:12–21

Blessed G, Tomlinson BE, Roth M (1968) The association between quantitative measures of dementia and of senile change in the cerebral grey matter of elderly subjects. Brit J Psychiatr 114:797–811

Chartier-Harlin MC, Crawford F, Houlden H, Warren A, Hughes D, Fidani L, Goate R, Rossor MN, Roques P, Hardy J, Mullan M (1991) Early-onset Alzheimer's disease caused by mutations at codon 717 of the beta-amyloid precursor protein gene. Nature 353:844–846

Cogan DG (1985) Visual disturbances with focal progressive dementing disease. Am J Ophthalmol 100:68–72

Crawford F, Hardy J, Mullan M, Goate A, Hughes D, Fidani L, Roques P, Rossor MN, Chartier-Hartlin MC (1991) Sequencing of exons 16 and 17 of the beta-amyloid precursor protein gene in 14 families with early onset Alzheimer's disease fails to reveal mutations in the beta-amyloid sequence. Neurosci Lett 133:1–2

Farrer LA, O'Sullivan DN, Cupples A, Growdon JH, Myers RH (1989) Assessment of genetic risk for Alzheimer's disease among 1st-degree relatives. Ann Neurol 25:485–493

Fitch N, Becker R, Heller A (1988) The inheritance of Alzheimer's disease: a new interpretation. Ann Neurol 23:14–19

Goate AM, Haynes AR, Owen MJ, Farrall M, James LA, Lai YC, Mullan MJ, Roques P, Rossor MN, Williamson R, Hardy JA (1989) Predisposing locus for Alzheimer's disease is on chromosome 21. Lancet 1:352–355

Goldgaber D, Lerman ML, McBride OW, Saffiotti V, Gajdusek DC (1987) Characterization and chromosomal localization of a cDNA encoding brain amyloid of Alzheimer's disease. Science 235:877–880

Haan J, Lanser JKB, Zijderveld I, van der Does IGF, Roos RAC (1990) Dementia in hereditary cerebral haemorhage with amyloidosis – Dutch type. Arch Neurol 47:965–967

Hansen L, Salmon D, Galasko D, Masliah E, Katzman R, DeTeresa R, Thal L, Pay MM, Hofstetter R, Klauber M, Rice V, Butters N, Alford M (1990) The Lewy Body variant of Alzheimer's disease: a clinical and pathologic entity. Neurology 40:1–8

Hardy J, Mullan M, Chartier-Harlin MC, Brown J, Goate A, Rossor MN, Collinge J, Roberts G, Luthert P, Lantos P, Naruse S, Kaneko K, Tsuji S, Miyatake T, Shimizu T, Kojima T, Nakano I, Yoshioka K, Sakaki Y, Miki T, Katsuya T, Ogihara T, Roses A, Pericak-Vance M, Haan J, Roos R, Lucotte C, David F (1991) Alzheimer's disease: a new nosology. Lancet 327:1342–1343

Heston LL, Mastri AR, Anderson VE, White J (1981) Dementia of the Alzheimer type: clinical genetics, natural history, and associated conditions. Arch Gen Psychiatr 38:1085–1090

Heston LL, Orr HT, Rich SS, White JA (1991) Linkage of an Alzheimer's disease susceptibility locus to markers on human chromosome 21. Am J Med Genet 40:449–453

Heyman A, Wilkinson WE, Hurtwitz BJ (1983) Alzheimer's disease: genetic aspects and associated clinical disorder. Ann Neurol 14:507–515

Huff FJ, Auerbach J, Chakravarti A, Boller F (1988) Risk of dementia in relatives of patients with Alzheimer's disease. Neurology 38:786–790

Jagust WJ, Davies P, Tiller-Borich JK, Reed BR (1990) Focal Alzheimer's disease. Neurology 40:14–19

Kang J, Lemaire HG, Unterbeck A, Salbaum JM, Masters CL, Grzeschik K-H, Multhaup G, Beyreuther K, Muller-Hill B (1987) The precursor of Alzheimer's disease amyloid A4 protein resembles a cell surface receptor. Nature 325:733–736

Karlinsky H, Madrick J, Ridgley J, Berg JM, Becker RC, Bergson C, Hodgkinson S, Percy M, McClachlan D (1991) A familiy with multiple instances of definite, probable and possible early onset Alzheimer's disease. Br J Psychiatr 159:524–530

Khachaturian ZS (1985) Diagnosis of Alzheimer's disease. Arch Neurol 42:1097–1105

Kirshner HS, Webb WG, Kelly MP, Wells CE (1984) Language disturbance. An initial symptom of cortical degenerations and dementia. Arch Neurol 41:491–496

Lantos PL, Luthert PJ, Hanger D, Anderton BH, Mullan M, Rossor MN (1992) Familial Alzheimer's disease with the amyloid precursor protein 717 mutation and sporadic Alzheimer's disease have the same cytoskeletal pathology. Neurosci Lett 137:221–224

Lowenberg K, Waggoner R (1934) Familial organic psychosis (Alzheimer's type). Arch Neurol Psychiatr 31:737–754

Martin JJ, Gheuens J, Bruyland M (1991) Early onset Alzheimer's disease in two large Belgian families. Neurology 41:62–68

Mayeux R, Stern Y, Spanton S (1985) Heterogeneity in dementia of the Alzheimer type: evidence of subgroups. Neurology 35:453–461

Mann DMA, Jones D, Snowden JS, Neary D, Hardy J (1992) Pathological changes in the brain of a patient with familial Alzheimer's disease having a missense mutation at codon 717 in the amyloid precursor protein gene. Neursoci Lett 137:225–228

McKhann G, Drachman D, Folstein M, Katzman R, Price D, Stradlan EM (1984) Clinical diagnosis of Alzheimer's disease. Neurology 34:939–944

Megendorfer F (1925) Über familiengeschichtliche Untersuchungen bei arteriosklerotischer und seniler Demenz. Zentralbl Neurol Psychiatr 40:359

Mohs RC, Breitner JCS, Silverman JM, Davis KL (1987) Alzheimer's disease. Morbid risk among first degree relatives approximates 50% by 90 years of age. Arch Gen Psychiatr 44:405–408

Mullan M, Tsuji S, Miki T et al (1992) Clinical and pathological comparison of Alzheimer's disease in pedigrees with the codon 717 Val→ Ile mutation in the amyloid precursor protein gene. (submitted)

Murrell J, Farlow M, Ghetti B, Benson MD (1991) A mutation in the amyloid precursor protein associated with hereditary Alzheimer's disease. Science 254:97–98

Nee LE, Polinsky R, Eldridge R (1983) A family with histologically confirmed Alzheimer's disease. Arch Neurol 40:203–208

Nee LE, Eldridge R, Sunderland T, Thomas CB, Katz D, Thompson KE, Weingartner H, Weiss H, Julian C, Cohen R (1987) Dementia of the Alzheimer type: clinical and family study of 22 twin pairs. Neurology 16:359–363

Pericak-Vance MA, Bebout JL, Gaskell PC Jr., Yamaoka LH, Hung W-Y, Alberts MJ, Walker AP, Bartlett RJ, Haynes CA, Welsh KA, Earl NL, Heyman A, Clark Cam, Roses AD (1991) Linkage studies in familial Alzheimer's disease: evidence for chromosome 19 linkage. Am J Human Genet 48:1034–1150

Pro YD, Smith CH, Sumi SM (1980) Presenile Alzheimer's disease: amyloid plaques in the cerebellum. Neurology 30:820–825

Schellenberg GD, Bird TD, Wijsman EM, Moore DK, Boehnke M, Bryant EM, Lampe TH, Nochlin D, Sumi SM, Deeb SS, Beyreuther K, Martin GM (1988) Absence of linkage of chromosome marker 21q21 markers to familial Alzheimer's disease. Science 241:1507–1510

Schellenberg GD, Anderson L, O'Dahl S, Wisjman EM, Sadovnick AD, Ball MJ, Larson EB, Kukull WA, Martin GM, Roses AD, Bird TD (1991) APP_{717}, APP_{693} and PRIP gene mutations are rare in Alzheimer's disease. Am J Human Genet 49:511–517

Schottky J (1932) Über Prasenile Verblodungen. Z Neurol Psychol 140:333–397

St George-Hyslop P, Tanzi R, Polinsky R, Haines JL, Nee L, Watkins PC, Myers RH, Feldman RG, Pollen D, Drachmann D, Growdon J, Bruni A, Foncin J-F, Salmon D, Frommelt P, Amaducci L, Sorbi S, Piacentini S, Stewart GD, Hobbs WJ, Conneally PM, Gusella JF (1987) The genetic defect causing familial Alzheimer's disease maps on chromosome 21. Science 235:885–890

St George-Hyslop PH, Haines JL, Farrer LA, Polinsky R, Van Broeckhoven C, Goate A, Crapper McLachlan DR, Orr H, Bruni AC, Sorbi S, Rainero I, Foncin JF, Pollen D, Cantu J-M, Tupler R, Voskresenskaya N, Mayeux R, Growdon J, Fried VA, Myers RH, Nee L, Backhovens H, Martin J-J, Rossor M, Owen MJ, Mullan M, Percy ME, Karlinsky K, Rich S, Heston L, Montesi M, Mortilla M, Nacmias N, Gusella JF (1990) Genetic linkage studies suggest that Alzheimer's disease is not a single homogeneous disorder. Nature 347:194–197

Tanzi RE, Gusella JF, Watkins PC, Bruns GAP, St George-Hyslop P, Van Keuren ML, Patterson D, Pagan S, Kurnit DM, Neve RL (1987a) Amyloid beta protein gene: cDNA, mRNA distribution and genetic linkage near the Alzheimer locus. Science 235:880–884

Tanzi RE, St George-Hyslop PH, Haines JL, Polinsky RY, Nee L, Foncin J-F, Neve RL, McClatchey AI, Conneally PM, Gusella JF (1987b) The genetic defect in familial Alzheimer's disease is not tightly linked to the amyloid beta-protein gene. Nature 329:156–157

Tyrrell PJ, Sawle GV, Ibanez V, Bloomfield PM, Leenders KL, Frackowiak RSJ, Rossor MN (1990) Clinical and PET studies in the "Extrapyramidal syndrome" of dementia of the Alzheimer type. Neurol 47:1318–1323

Van Broeckhoven C, Genthe AM, Vandenberghe A, Hosthemke B, Backhovens H, Raey-maekers P, Van Hul W, Wehnert A, Gheuns J, Cras P, Bruyland M, Martin JJ, Salbaum M, Multhaup G, Masters CL, Beyreuther K, Gurling HMD, Mullan MJ, Holland A, Barton A, Irving N, Williamson R, Richards SJ, Hardy JA (1987) Failure of familial Alzheimer's disease to segregate with the A4-amyloid gene in several European families. Nature 329:153–155

Van Duijn CM, Van Broeckhoven C, Hardy JA, Goate AM, Rossor MN, Vandenberghe A, Martin J-J, Hofman A and Mullan MJ (1991) Evidence for allelic heterogeneity in familial early-onset Alzheimer's disease. Br J of Psychiatr 158:471–474

Molecular Genetic Evidence for Etiologic Heterogeneity of Alzheimer's Disease

P. H. St George-Hyslop, D. R. Crapper McLachlan, J. L. Haines,
A. Bruni, J.-F. Foncin, W. Lukiw, M. P. Montesi, M. Mortilla,
L. Pinessi, R. J. Polinsky, D. Pollen, I. Rainero, E. Rogaev,
S. Sorbi, R. Tanzi, R. Tupler, and G. Vaula

In the last several years considerable evidence has accumulated which argues that Alzheimer's disease (AD) is etiologically heterogeneous. In particular, molecular genetic studies of pedigrees with familial Alzheimer's disease (FAD) have provided quite convincing evidence that different primary events (defects in different genes) are capable of causing the same general disease phenotype associated with AD (i.e., adult onset progressive dementia accompanied by the characteristic neuropathologic features of neurofibrillary degeneration and amyloid deposits, etc.). This review will examine some of the molecular genetic evidence for etiologic heterogeneity.

Genetic Linkage Studies Suggest That FAD is Heterogeneous

It is now well recognized that patients with trisomy 21 (Down's Syndrome – DS) who survive beyond the age of 40 years almost universally have the neuropathological attributes of AD on post-mortem examination and may also frequently show ante-mortem, clinically apparent dementia. These observations suggest that chromosome 21 may harbour one or more genes involved in the pathogenesis of AD. Genetic linkage studies using polymorphic molecular probes from chromosome 21 by this group, and subsequently by other groups, confirmed that the FAD trait, and thus the FAD gene in at least some pedigrees cosegregated with markers from the proximal long arm of chromosome 21 (St George Hyslop et al. 1987). However, similar linkage studies by two other groups – one investigating a large group of pedigrees enriched in pedigrees with a later age of onset (> 65 years), and the other investigating a group of pedigrees enriched in pedigrees of Volga German origin – failed to detect co-segregation between FAD and the same chromosome 21 markers when their overall data were examined (Schellenberg et al., 1988; Pericak-Vance et al., 1988).

These conflicting observations initially lead to uncertainty as to whether the initial linkage studies were in error, or whether the apparent disparity reflected etiologic heterogeneity (i.e., only some of the pedigrees were linked to chromsome 21 whereas other pedigrees harboured genetic defects on other chromosomes or represented familial clustering of a mixed genetic-environmental or non-genetic cause). This uncertainty was effectively resolved,however, by the investigation of a larger data set which included pedigrees of diverse ethnic origins and with different phenotypic expressions of FAD (age of onset ranging

F. Boller et al. (Eds.)
Heterogeneity of Alzheimer's Disease
© Springer-Verlag Berlin Heidelberg 1992

from 35 to 89 years). Analysis of this data set clearly revealed that evidence for co-segregation of FAD with genetic markers from chromosome 21 was derived predominantly from pedigrees with a pre-senile onset of FAD ($\leq$ 65 years), whereas pedigrees with senile onset FAD ($>$ 65 years) in general gave negative lod scores. The difference between the linkage data provided by the pre-senile onset and the senile onset pedigrees was both statistically significant and robust over several different methods of analysis. This observation clearly supported the hypothesis that FAD was etiologically heterogeneous, and provided an explanation for the apparant disparity between the initial linkage results from different groups (St George-Hyslop et al., 1990).

At this juncture, two new questions arose:

1. what is the identity of the gene or genes on chromosome 21 causing pre-senile onset FAD, and
2. what is the chromosomal location or locations of the FAD genes causing FAD that are not linked to chromosome 21?

Subsequent Linkage Studies on Chromosomes other than Chromosome 21

Recent work by Roses et al. in their late onset pedigrees has provided tentative evidence of a late onset FAD locus on chromosome 19q (Pericak-Vance et al., 1991). Intriguingly, an allelic association but no close genetic linkage had been previously reported between FAD and certain alleles of the APO CII gene on chromosome 19q by Schellenberg et al. (1992). While the relationship remains unclear between the observations of allelic association without linkage in one study and of both linkage and allelic association in the second study, it is obvious that additional investigation of chromosome 19 in FAD pedigrees will be required.

To this end, we have tested a series of closely linked chromosome 19 markers. (Bcl3; Na K ATPase; D19S47; D19S49; CEA, and D19S13) which straddle the region of chromosome 19 identified by Roses et al. Unfortunately, despite a considerable effort, the results in our pedigrees have been largely uninformative. The early onset pedigrees as a group have provided negative results, although a few early onset pedigrees have given small positive lod scores ($\hat{z} < +2.00$) for some of these markers. The late onset pedigrees as a group have provided weakly positive scores which clearly do not exclude linkage but do not provide independent proof of linkage. Because most of our pedigrees yielded indeterminate scores we were also unable to obtain statistically significant evidence for or against heterogeneity. However, although our data *per se* has not provided definitive results to date, this data can still be used as part of a larger data set to further investigate the role of chromosome 19 in the pathogenesis of FAD. Investigations are now under way with Roses et al. to test various hypotheses including the tempting speculation that the FAD trait in some pedigrees may in fact arise from the cooperative effect of two independent loci (see the chapter by Roses et al. elsewhere in volume).

Further Analysis of Chromosome 21

Direct inspection of the pedigrees specific lod scores for the subset of pedigrees with a presenile onset described above, clearly argue that not all pedigrees with an early onset are linked to chromosome 21. Furthermore, the multipoint linkage analyses using the markers D21S13/S16 (centromeric) and D21S1/S11 (telomeric), and the LINKAGE (ver 3.0) computer program provided a bimodal distribution of likelihoods, with one peak $\hat{Z} = +5.03$) centromeric to D21S13/S16, and a second peak ($\hat{Z} = +5.00$) located telomeric to D21S1/S11. While we were unable to statistically prove that this bimodal distribution of likelihoods reflected the existence of two FAD loci on chromosome 21, it was abundantly obvious that the telomeric peak overlay the location of the amyloid precursor protein (APP) gene (St George-Hyslop et al., 1990).

The APP gene was an obvious candidate gene for the site of an FAD mutation. However, we had previously observed recombination events between the FAD trait and the APP gene in our largest pedigrees, including the FAD4 pedigree, which gives highly suggestive lod scores ($z \geq +2.00$) for several markers on the proximal long arm of chromosome 21 (e.g., D21S13/S16 and D21S59). These recombination events, and similar events reported by Hardy and van Broeckhoven, suggested that mutations in APP were unlikely to be found at least in our pedigrees (van Broeckhoven et al., 1987; Tanzi et al. 1987). However, Hardy and colleagues had two pedigrees which had not shown recombination events with APP, and in fact had shown substantial positive evidence for cosegregation with APP. Direct sequencing of the APP gene in these pedigrees had been suggested at the 1989 Niigata meeting and the 1990 Toronto AD meeting (D. Selkoe, S. Prusiner and others). A further impetus for sequencing the APP gene in these pedigrees was the discovery by Levy et al. (1990) of a mutation in exon 17 of the APP gene at codon 693 in pedigrees with Hereditary Cerebral Hemorrhage with Angiopathy – Dutch Type (HCHWA-D). Bearing these suggestions in mind, Hardy and colleagues subsequently initiated DNA sequencing studies in their pedigrees using the PCR protocols of Levy et al., and were able to demonstrate a new missense mutation in the same exon of the APP gene (Val $\rightarrow$ Ile substitution at codon 717) in both of the non-recombinant pedigrees) (Goate et al., 1991).

Sequencing Studies on the APP Gene

The observation of missense mutations in the APP gene of at least two FAD pedigrees raised the question as to whether misdiagnosis, non-paternity or other technical errors may have accounted for some of the recombination events previously observed between APP and the FAD gene in pedigrees showing evidence of co-segregation with other chromosome 21 markers. To address this question, we re-evaluated the diagnosis, the paternity, and DNA typings of several critical individuals who defined genetic recombination between FAD and APP in our previous studies. None of the recombination events previously observed was refuted on this re-analysis. Subsequent to our initial linkage studies we had acquired several smaller pedigrees which did not show recombination with APP, but also did not show strong evidence of linkage to chromosome 21 or APP ($z > +1.00$). The existence of a mutation in APP in these pedigrees could not be excluded on solely genetic grounds. Furthermore, it was theoretically still possible that mutations might have occurred in the APP gene in our recombinant pedigrees, but that this possibility might have been obscured by recombination events within the APP gene itself. Such intragenic recombination events have been observed in large genes like the Duchenne Muscular Dystrophy (DMD) gene, although the DMD gene is considerably larger than the APP gene (2 Mbases compared to 150 Kbases). We decided to address the possibility that APP might be the site of the mutation in the smaller pedigrees, and to address the possibility of erroneous exclusion of APP due to intragenic recombination events, by directly searching our pedigrees for mutations in the APP gene (Tanzi et al., 1992).

The entire coding sequence (exons 1–18 inclusive), the intron-exon boundaries, and the 3′ untranslated sequence were investigated by direct sequencing of PCR products in two large pedigrees (FAD1, which shows no substantial evidence of linkage to chromosome 21, and FAD4, which shows positive but subsignificant evidence of linkage to chromosome 21). A sequence difference (C → T substitution) was noted at nucleotide 104 (codon 34) of exon 4 in an affected member of FAD4 (Vaula et al., submitted for publication). Further studies revealed that:

1. this mutation was unlikely to be pathogenic because the mutation would not be predicted to change the encoded amino acid,
2. the mutation was inherited from the uanffected parent, and
3. the mutation was also present in two elderly unaffected siblings, but
4. the mutation was not present in four other affected family members. No other mutations were detected in any other exon of either FAD1 or FAD4 (Tanzi et al., 1992).

The investigation of the remaining pedigrees was confined to exons 16 and 17 and their 5′ and 3′ intron-exon boundaries. Twenty-five other pedigrees were investigated by direct sequencing of PCR products from exon 16 and 17. Twenty more pedigrees were investigated by BcII cleavage of the exon 17 PCR product to screen for the Val → Ile mutation at codon 717 and by cleavage with MaeIII to screen for the Ala → Val mutation at codon 713. Eighty-one cases of AD without known family history were screened for somatic mutations in exon 17 by PCR amplification from frozen postmortem brain of patients dying with neuropathologically proven AD. Of the 126 independent AD/FAD cases examined, only one case (the 124th case investigated) showed a mutation in exon 17 (Karlinksy et al., 1992). No mutations were detected in exon 16. This observation clearly argues that FAD and sporadic AD are only rarely associated with mutations in APP. Similar observations have been made by several other groups (Schellenberg et al., 1991; Van Duijn et al., 1991).

Characterization of a Single Pedigree with an APP$_{717}$ Mutation

The single pedigree (TOR3) detected in the screening of 126 independent AD cases is a nuclear pedigrees that emigrated to Canada from the British Isles approximately 200 years ago. The FAD trait manifests in the fifth decade (47.6 ± 3.0 yrs) and appears to segregate as an autosomal dominant trait through the three generations for which reliable medical or family records are available. Neuropathologic confirmation of antemortem clinically diagnosed FAD has been obtained for two members. Three members of this pedigrees are currently living and affected by FAD. Neuropathology confirmation of the absence of AD was available for a single elderly unaffected pedigree member who died at more than five standard deviations beyond mean age-of-onset in this family, indicating that this individual must be considered as an obligate unaffected member.

Sequencing of the APP gene in this pedigree revealed the presence of a missense mutation (G → A) at position 2150 in exon 17 (APP$_{770}$ isoform), which would be predicted to cause a Val → Ile substitution at codon 717. This mutation co-segregated perfectly with the FAD trait in this family, and was not present in the obligate unaffected pedigree member ($\hat{Z} = +3.45$ at $\hat{\Theta} = 0.00$) (Karlinsky et al., 1992).

The clinical phenotype of the living affected members has been documented prospectively from a very early stage in the illness, and will be presented in detail elsewhere. The neuropathologic attributes of the disease phenotype in the TOR3 pedigree are typical of AD (abundant neuritic plaques, neurofibrillary degeneration, neuronal loss, mild amyloid angiopathy) but lack some of the features observed in other pedigrees with APP mutations, such as Lewy Bodies or angiopathy accompanied by clinical sequelae such as stroke or cerebral hemorrhage. Quantitative neuropathologic studies are currently underway.

Significance of the APP$_{717}$ Mutation

At the current time the most straightforward explanation for the role of the APP$_{717}$ mutation in the pathogenesis of AD is that it is causative as postulated by Hardy et al. (Goate et al. 1991). However, two additional observations must be considered before alternate explanations are completely rejected. First, it would appear that there is no consistent phenotype amongst the published pedigrees with APP$_{717}$ mutations except that they ALL have had a presenile onset of symptoms. Second, the observations by Roses et al. (this volume) that their pedigree with an APP$_{717}$ mutation also shows strong but subsignificant evidence of cosegregation with markers from chromosome 19q raises the possibility that the APP$_{717}$ mutation could be involved in the timing of onset of symptoms (i.e., it may be epistatic to other genes or environmental causes). Obviously, the best evidence to support such a hypothesis would be the discovery of predigrees in which the mutation is not present in all affected members, and the disease has a later onset in members without the mutation. In the APP$_{717}$/FAD pedigree described by Roses et al. (this volume), there are two distant family members affected by AD but who both lack the APP_{717} mutation and who both have a later age of onset (after 65 years compared to less than 50 years for the APP_{717} carrying affected members). A similar observations has also been made by van Broeckhoven and colleagues who have described a pedigree with familial presenile dementia or cerebral hemorrhage associated with a mutation at codon 692 in exon 17. One member of this family has a dementia with a slightly later age of onset (61 years compared to less than 54 years) but lacks the mutation observed in the other affected pedigrees members (Hendricks et al., 1992). These observations raise the tantalizing but as yet unanswerable question – are these non-mutant affected pedigree members simply sporadic phenocopies or do they reflect a more complicated relationship between mutations in the APP gene and the disease phenotype?

It is of note that the Val → Ile APP_{717} mutation has been described in 10 pedigrees to date, but that only single cases of the Val → Gly and Val → Phe mutations have been described (Hardy, this volume). The explanation for this observations is unclear. It is also noteworthy that of the 10 pedigrees with the Val → Ile mutation five have been of Japanese origin and four have been of British origin. To date, this mutation has been absent from pedigrees of Italian, French/French Canadian, and Ashkenazi Jewish origin that have been screened by this group. The observation of clustering of cases on two island nations argues for the existence of a common founder for at least some but probably not all of the cases in each country. However, it is probably unlikely that the Japanese and the British cases share common founders. While the possibility of a founder effect in each population should be relatively easy to test, a note of caution needs to be interjected concerning the use of hypervariable tandem repeat polymorphisms (dinucleotide or higher order repeats) as genetic markers in linkage disequilibrium studies, because of reports that these markers may spontenously alter the number of tandem repeats by a mechanism other than genetic recombination at a frequency of between 0.0045/locus/gamete and 0.05/locus/gamete.

The Current Status of Presenile Onset Pedigrees without Mutations in APP

At least two of the largest and best characterized pedigrees with presenile onset FAD (FAD4 and AD/A) have not yet been found to harbour mutations in the APP gene yet continue to display positive but subsignificant lod scores ($\hat{Z}$ approximately + 2.00) for one or more markers elsewhere on the proximal long arm of chromosome 21 (St George-Hyslop et al. 1990). The significance of these observations remain to be determined, but at face value they would seem to indicate the existence of another putative FAD locus on chromosome 21, perhaps having a long range cis-acting effect on the expression of APP itself. This suggestion is supported by the observation of a bimodal distribution of lod scores for the presenile onset pedigrees in our previous analysis noted earlier, with one peak (z = + 5.03) located centromeric to D21S13/S16, and one peak (z = + 5.00) being located telomeric to D21S1/S11 (i.e., near APP). However, it is also possible that these results may simply represent statistical artifacts. Indeed, Hardy et al. have stated that the discovery of mutations in two of the presenile onset pedigrees contributing to the overall positive lod scores for chromosome 21 negatives any need to invoke the existence of other genes elsewhere on chromosome 21 (Crawford et al., 1991). Resolution of this dilemma will require investigation of these pedigrees both with additional markers from chromosome 21 and with markers from other chromosomes.

References

Crawford F, Hardy J, Mullan M, Goate A, Hughes D, Fidani L, Roques P, Rossor M, Chartier-Harlin MC (1991) Sequencing of exons 16 and 17 of the β-amyloid precursor protein gene in families with early onset Alzheimer's disease fails to reveal mutations in the β-amyloid sequence. Neurosci Lett 133:1–2

Goate A, Chartier-Harlin MC, Mullan M, Brown J, Crawford F, Fidani L, Giuffra L, Haynes A, Irving N, James L, Mant R, Newton P, Rooke K, Roques P, Talbot C, Pericak-Vance M, Roses A, Williamson R, Rossor M, Owen M, Hardy J (1991) Segregation of a missense mutation in the amyloid precursor protein gene with familial Alzheimer's disease. Nature 349:704–706

Hendriks L, van Duijn CM, Cras P et al (1992) in press

Karlinksy H, Vaula G, St George-Hyslop PH et al (1992) Molecular genetic and prospective phenotypic characterization of a pedigree segregating familial Alzheimer's disease and a mutation in codon 717 of the β-amyloid precursor protein gene. Neurology, in press

Levy E, Carman MD, Fernandez-Madrid IJ, Power MD, Lieberburg I, Van Duinen SG, Bots GTAM, Luyendijk W, Frangione B (1990) Mutation of the Alzheimer's disease amyloid gene in hereditary cerebral hemorrhage – Dutch type. Science 248:1124–1226

Pericak-Vance MA, Yamaoka LH, Haynes CS, Speer MC, Haines JL, Gaskell PC, Hung W-Y, Clark CM, Heyman AL, Trofatter JA, Eisenmenger JP, Gilbert JR, Lee JE, Alberts MJ, Dawson DV, Bartlett RJ, Earl NL, Siddique T, Vance JM, Conneally PM, Roses AD (1988) Genetic linkage studies in Alzheimer's disease families. Exp Neurol 102:271–279

Pericak-Vance MA, Bedout JL, Gaskell PC, Yamaoka LH, Hung W-Y, Alberts MJ, Walker AP, Bartlett RJ, Haynes CA, Welsh KA, Earl NL, Heyman A, Clark Cam, Roses AD (1991) Linkage studies in familial Alzheimer disease – evidence for chromosome 19 linkage. Am J Hum Genet 48:1034–1050

Schlellenberg GD, Bird TD, Wijsman EM, Moore DK, Boehnke M, Bryant EM, Lampe TH, Nochlin D, Sumi SM, Deeb SS, Beyreuther K, Martin GM (1988) Absence of linkage of chromosome 21q21 markers to familial Alzheimer disease. Science 241:1507–1510

Schellenberg GD, Boehnke M, Wijsman EM, Moore DK, Martin GM, Bird TD (1992) Genetic association and linkage analysis of the apolipoprotein CII locus and familial. Alzheimer's disease. Ann Neurol 31:223–227

Schellenberg GD, Anderson L, O'Dahl S, Wijsman EM, Sadovnick AD, Ball MJ, Larson EB, Kukull WA, Martin GM, Roses AD, Bird TD (1991) APP_{717}, APP_{693} and PrP mutations are rare in Alzheimer's disease. Am J Hum Genet 49:511–517

St George-Hyslop PH, Tanzi RE, Polinsky RJ, Haines JL, Nee L, Watkins PC, Myers RH, Feldman RG, Pollen D, Drachmann D, Growdon J, Bruni A, Foncin J-F, Salmon D, Frommelt P, Amaducci L, Sorbi S, Piacentini S, Stewart GD, Hobbs WJ, Conneally PM, Gusella JF (1987) The genetic defect causing familial Alzheimer disease maps on chromosome 21. Science 235:885–889

St George-Hyslop PH, Haines JL, Farrer LA, Polinsky R, Van Broeckhoven C, Goate A, Crapper McLachlan DR, Orr H, Bruni AC, Sorbi S, Rainero I, Foncin JF, Pollen D, Cantu J-M, Tupler R, Voskresenskaya N, Mayeux R, Growdon J, Fried VA, Myers RH, Nee L, Backhovens H, Martin J-J, Rossor M, Owen MJ, Mullan M, Percy ME, Karlinsky K, Rich S, Heston L, Montesi M, Mortilla M, Nacmias N, Gusella JF (1990) Genetic linkage studies suggest that Alzheimer's disease is not a single homogeneous disorder. Nature 347:194–197

Tanzi RE, St George-Hyslop PH, Haines JL, Polinsky RJ, Nee L, Foncin J-F, Neve RL, McClatchey AI, Conneally PM, Gusella JG (1987) The genetic defect in familial Alzheimer's disease is not tightly linked to the β-amyloid precursor gene. Nature 331, 528–530

Tanzi RE, Vaula G, Romano D, St George-Hyslop PH (1992) Assessment of amyloid β-protein precursor gene mutations in a large set of familial and sporadic Alzheimer Disease cases. Am J Human Genet, in press

van Broeckhoven C, Genthe CA, Vandenberghe B, Hosthemke B, Backhovens H, Raeymaekers P, Van Hul W, Wehnert A, Gheuns J, Cras P, Bruyland M, Martin JJ, Salbaum M, Multhaup G, Masters CL, Beyreuther K, Gurling HMD, Mullan MJ, Holland A, Barton A, Irving N, Williamson R, Richards SJ, Hardy JA (1987) Failure of familial Alzheimer's disease to segregate with the A-4 amyloid gene in several European families. Nature 329:153–154

van Duijn CM, Hendriks L, Cruts M, Hardy J, Hofman A, van Broeckoven C (1991) Amyloid precursor protein gene mutation in early onset Alzheimer's disease. Lancet 337:978

Alzheimer's Disease:
many Aetiologies; one Pathogenesis

J. Hardy

Summary

Recent genetic studies have clearly shown that Alzheimer's disease (AD) has several aetiologies. Some cases have defined mutations in the β-amyloid precursor protein (APP) gene, others do not. Persons with Down's syndrome presumably get AD because they constitutively overexpress APP. Despite these differences in aetiology, all cases seem to have similar clinical and pathological features. The simplest explanation of the fact that there are several aetiologies, but a single pathology, is that a pathological cascade occurs which can be triggered in several ways. It is not yet clear whether there are small clinical and pathological differences between cases with different aetiologies.

Introduction

The pathology of AD is complex. There are extracellular neuritic plaques, largely consisting of deposits of a peptide β-amyloid (Masters et al., 1985; Glenner and Wong, 1984), intracellular neurofibrillary tangles largely consisting of over-phosphorylated tau (Lee et al., 1991) and cell loss (Mann et al., 1987).

Pathological investigations have not allowed this complex pathology to be ordered, i.e., it has not been possible to determine whether one aspect of the pathology comes first and causes the others, or whether they are independent sequellae of another primary event. Studies on Down's syndrome have, however, suggested that β-amyloid deposition is an early event in the process (Mann and Esiri, 1989).

Genetics of AD

Occasionally, early onset AD segregates as an autosomal dominant disorder (reviewed in St. George-Hyslop et al., 1989). In one such family, we used molecular genetic techniques to identify a point mutation at codon 717, causing a valine to isoleucine change in APP (Goate et al., 1991). This mutation has subsequently been detected in several other families with early-onset AD, but not in the general population, in sporadic cases of AD or in late-onset cases of

F. Boller et al. (Eds.)
Heterogeneity of Alzheimer's Disease
© Springer-Verlag Berlin Heidelberg 1992

AD, whether familial or sporadic (Goate et al., 1991; Naruse et al., 1991; Yoshioka et al., 1991; Hardy et al., 1991). Thus, this mutation is a rare cause of AD (Goate et al., 1991; van Duijn et al., 1991b). Subsequently, two other mutations at codon 717 have been described in single families: the first, changing valine to phenylalanine (Murrell et al., 1991), and the second, changing valine to glycine (Chartier-Harlin et al., 1991b). It is not yet clear whether mutations at other sites in the APP gene also lead to AD; however, these results clearly demonstrate that hereditary, early-onset AD is allelically heterogeneous (van Duijn et al., 1991c).

However, genetic linkage analysis clearly shows that there are many families, probably the majority, in which the APP gene does not segregate with early-onset AD (Tanzi et al., 1987; Van Broeckhoven et al., 1987; Schellenberg et al., 1988, 1991). This contention is supported by the observation that the majority of families with early-onset AD do not appear to have mutations in this gene (Chartier-Harlin et al., 1991a; Crawford et al., 1991). Thus, early-onset, familial AD also shows locus heterogeneity (Schellenberg et al., 1988, 1991; St. George-Hyslop et al., 1990). Genetic analysis has not yet allowed determination of the location of the non-APP locus; indeed there may be more than one other locus.

The β-Amyloid Cascade Hypothesis of AD

The majority of cases of AD, however, do not seem to have a simple genetic aetiology. Even within the early-onset group, most cases do not have a family history (van Duijn et al., 1991a). Within the late-onset group, most cases are not familial, and those that are show a pattern of "inheritance" not consistent with autosomal dominance (van Duijn et al. 1991a; Farrer et al. 1990, 1991). Thus, AD must also show aetiological heterogeneity.

As yet, there are no other proven aetiologies for AD; however, the fact that mutations in APP are one cause strongly suggests that APP mismetabolism and β-amyloid deposition are the causes of the entire pathology in those cases with mutations. Constitutive overexpression of APP is likely to be the cause of AD in Down's syndrome (Hardy and Allsop, 1991; Rumble et al., 1989). By analogy with AD in families with APP mutations and with AD in Down's syndrome, it would seem most likely that APP mismetabolism is an early event in the pathogenesis of other cases of the disease (Hardy and Allsop, 1991). Partial confirmation of this hypothesis has come from the recent report of transgenic animals who over-expressed a β-amyloid-containing construct and developed the full AD pathology (Kawabata et al., 1992).

Head Injury and AD

Dementia pugilistica is characterized by diffuse β-amyloid deposition, neurofibrillary tangles and neuronal loss (Roberts et al., 1990), and can thus be thought of as a form of AD caused by repeated blows to the head. Consistent with this simplistic notion is the observation that APP is up-regulated by head injury in animals and in man (Roberts et al., 1991; Kawarabayashi et al., 1991). Furthermore, epidemiological studies consistently identify head injury as a risk for developing AD (Mortimer et al., 1991). These observations suggest that, at least in some, perhaps genetically predisposed individuals, the pathological cascade can be triggered by head injury-induced, up-regulation of APP.

Are there Clinical Discriminators of AD Aetiology?

As it is clear from the above that there are several causes of AD, the immediate question is whether AD of different aetiologies has a subtly different pathological or clinical phenotype. At present, there is little evidence to address this issue and only incomplete statements can be given. These include:
1. Pathologically, AD in Down's syndrome appears very similar to AD in the general population (Mann et al., 1984).
2. Families with each APP mutation seem to have a consistent onset age (Hardy et al., 1991; van Duijn et al., 1991b); however, other families which do not have APP mutations also have similar onset ages (Crawford et al., 1991).
3. While families with APP mutations appear to have a relatively consistent presentation, not enough families with each mutation have yet been clinically and pathologically investigated to determine whether this consistency in presentation is family, or mutation, specific.
4. The clinical features of dementia pugilistica are clearly distinguishable from those of typical AD; however, dementia pugilistica is clearly an extreme example and is complicated in that there are causes of neuronal loss other than the AD pathology.

For these reasons, it is not yet possible to determine whether the variability in the clinical presentation of AD has aetiologic significance. If clinical or pathological discriminators of aetiology could be identified, it would be of enormous assistance in defining the other risk factors, both genetic and epigenetic, since one could determine the risk factors for each form separately. This approach would resemble the approach which has been so successfully applied to heart disease.

References

Chartier-Harlin MC, Crawford F, Hamandi K, Mullan M, Goate A, Backhovens H, Martin JJ, Van Broeckhoven C (1991a) Screening for the β-amyloid precursor protein mutation (APP:Val→Ile), in extended pedigrees with early onset Alzheimer's disease. Neurosci Lett 129:134–135

Chartier-Harlin MC, Crawford F, Houlden H, Warren A, Hughes D, Fidani L, Goate A, Rossor M, Roques P, Hardy J, Mullan M (1991b) Early onset Alzheimer's disease caused by mutations of codon 717 of the β-amyloid precursor protein gene. Nature 353:844–846

Crawford F, Hardy J, Mullan M, Goate A, Hughes D, Fidani L, Roques P, Rossor M, Chartier-Harlin MC (1991) Sequencing of exons 16 and 17 of the β-amyloid precursor protein gene in families with early onset Alzheimer's disease fails to reveal mutations in the β-amyloid sequence. Neurosci Lett 133:1–2

Farrer LA, Myers RH, Cupples LA, St. George-Hyslop PH, Bird TD, Rossor MN, Mullan MJ, Polinsky R, Nee L, Heston L, van Broeckoven C, Martin JJ, Crapper McLachlan D, Growdon JH (1990) Transmission and age-at-onset patterns in familial Alzheimer's disease: evidence for heterogeneity. Neurology 40:395–403

Farrer LA, Myers RH, Connor L, Cupples LA, Growdon JH (1991) Segregation analysis reveals evidence of a major gene for Alzheimer's disease. Am J Hum Genet 48:1026–1033

Glenner GG, Wong CW (1984) Alzheimer's disease: initial report of the purification and characterization of a novel cerebrovascular amyloid protein. Biochem Biophys Res Commun 120:885–890

Goate A, Chartier-Harlin MC, Mullan M, Brown J, Crawford F, Fidani L, Giuffra L, Haynes A, Irving N, James L, Mant R, Newton P, Rooke K, Roques P, Talbot C, Pericak-Vance M, Roses A, Williamson R, Rossor M, Owen M, Hardy J (1991) Segregation of a missense mutation in the amyloid precursor protein gene with familial Alzheimer's disease. Nature 349:704–706

Hardy J, Allsop D (1991) Amyloid deposition as the central event in the aetiology of Alzheimer's disease. Trends Pharmacol 12:383–388

Hardy J, Mullan M, Chartier-Harlin MC, Brown J, Goate A, Rossor M, Collinge J, Roberts G, Luthert P, Lantos P, Naruse S, Kaneko K, Tsuji S, Miyatake T, Shimizu T, Kojima T, Nakano I, Yoshioka K, Sakaki Y, Miki T, Katsuya T, Ogihara T, Roses A, Pericak-Vance M, Haan J, Roos R, Lucotte G, David F (1991) Molecular classification of Alzheimer's disease. Lancet 337:1342–1343

Kawabata S, Higgins GA, Gordon JW (1992) Amyloid plaques, neurofibrillary tangles and neuronal loss in brains of transgenic mice overexpressing a C-terminal fragment of human amyloid precursor protein. Nature, in press

Kawarabayashi T, Shoji M, Harigaya Y, Yamaguchi H, Hirai S (1991) Expression of APP in the early stage of brain damage. Brain Res 563:334–338

Lee VM, Balin BJ, Otvos LJ, Trojanowski JQ (1991) A68: a major subunit of paired helical filaments and derivatized forms of normal Tau. Science 251:675–678

Mann DM, Esiri MM (1989) The pattern of acquisition of plaques and tangles in the brains of patients under 50 years of age with Down's syndrome. J Neurol Sci 89:169–179

Mann DM, Yates PO, Marcyniuk B (1984) Alzheimer's presenile dementia, senile dementia of Alzheimer type and Down's syndrome in middle age form, an age related continuum of pathological changes. Neuropathol Appl Neurobiol 10:185–207

Mann DM, Yates PO, Marcyniuk B, Ravindra CR (1987) Loss of neurones from cortical and subcortical areas in Down's syndrome patients at middle age. Quantitative comparisons with younger Down's patients and patients with Alzheimer's disease. J Neurol Sci 80:79–89

Masters CL, Simms G, Weinman NA, Multhaup G, McDonald BL, Beyreuther K (1985) Amyloid plaque core protein in Alzheimer disease and Down syndrome. Proc Natl Acad Sci USA 82:4245–4249

Mortimer JA, van Duijn CM, Chandra V, Fratiglioni L, Graves AB, Heyman A, Jorm AF, Kokmen E, Kondo K, Rocca WA, Shalat SL, Soininen H, Hofman A (1991) Head trauma as a risk factor for Alzheimer's disease: A collaborative re-analysis of case-control studies. Int J Epidemiol 20 Suppl 2:S28–S35

Murrell J, Farlow M, Ghetti B, Benson M (1991) A mutation in the amyloid precursor protein associated with hereditary Alzheimer's disease. Science 254:97–99

Naruse S, Igarashi S, Kobayashi H, Aoki K, Inuzuka T, Kaneko K, Shimizu T, Iihara K, Kojima T, Miyatake T, Tsuji S (1991) Mis-sense mutation Val→Ile in exon 17 of amyloid precursor protein gene in Japanese familial Alzheimer's disease. Lancet 337:978–979

Roberts GW, Allsop D, Bruton C (1990) The occult aftermath of boxing. J Neurol Neurosurg Psych 53:373–378

Roberts GW, Gentleman SM, Lynch A, Graham DI (1991) β/A4 amyloid protein deposition in brain after head trauma. Lancet 338:1422–1423

Rumble B, Retallack R, Hilbich C, Simms G, Multhaup G, Martins R, Hockey A, Montgomery P, Beyreuther K, Masters CL (1989) Amyloid A4 protein and its precursor in Down's synrome and Alzheimer's disease. N Engl J Med 320:1446–1452

Schellenberg GD, Bird TD, Wijsman EM, Moore DK, Boehnke M, Bryant EM, Lampe TH, Nochlin D, Sumi SM, Deeb SS, Beyreuther K, Martin GM (1988) Absence of linkage of chromosome 21q21 markers to familial Alzheimer's disease. Science 241:1507–1510

Schellenberg GD, Pericak Vance MA, Wijsman EM, Moore DK, Gaskell PCJ, Yamaoka LA, Bebout JL, Anderson L, Welsh KA, Clark CM, Martin GM, Roses AD, Bird TD (1991) Linkage analysis of familial Alzheimer disease, using chromosome 21 markers. Am J Human Genet 48:563–583

St George-Hyslop PH, Haines JL, Farrer LA, Polinsky R, Van Broeckhoven C, Goate A, McLachlan DR, Orr H, Bruni AC, Sorbi S, Rainero I, Foncin JF, Pollen D, Cantu J-M, Tupler R, Voskresenskaya N, Mayeux R, Growdon J, Fried VA, Myers RH, Nee L, Backhovens H, Martin J-J, Rossor M, Owen MJ, Mullan M, Percy ME, Karlinsky K, Rich S, Heston L, Montesi M, Mortilla M, Nacmias N, Gusella JF (1990) Genetic linkage studies suggest that Alzheimer's disease is not a single homogeneous disorder. FAD Collaborative Study Group. Nature 347:194–197

St George-Hyslop PH, Myers RH, Haines JL, Farrer LA, Tanzi RE, Abe K, James MF, Conneally PM, Polinsky RJ, Gusella JF (1989) Familial Alzheimer's disease: progress and problems. Neurobiol Aging 10:417–427

Tanzi RE, St George-Hyslop PH, Haines JL, Polinsky RJ, Nee L, Foncin JF, Neve RL, McClatchey AI, Conneally PM, Gusella JF (1987) The genetic defect in familial Alzheimer's disease is not tightly linked to the amyloid beta-protein gene. Nature 329:156–157

van Broeckhoven C, Genthe AM, Vandenberghe A, Horsthemke B, Backhovens H, Raeymaekers P, Van Hul W, Wehnert A, Gheuens J, Cras P, Bruyland M, Martin JJ, Salbaum M, Multhaup G, Masters CL, Beyreuther K, Gurling HMD, Mullan MJ, Holland A, Barton A, Irving N, Williamson R, Richards SJ, Hardy JA (1987) Failure of familial Alzheimer's disease to segregate with the A4-amyloid gene in several European families. Nature 329:153–155

van Duijn CM, Clayton D, Chandra V, Fratiglioni L, Graves AB, Heyman A, Jorm AF, Kokmen E, Kondo K, Mortimer JA, Rocca WA, Shalat SL, Soininen H, Hofman A (1991a) Familial aggregation of Alzheimer's disease and related disorders: A collaborative re-analysis of case-control studies. Int J Epidemiol 20 Suppl 2:S13–S20

van Duijn CM, Hendriks L, Cruts M, Hardy JA, Hofman A, van Broeckhoven CM (1991b) Amyloid precursor protein gene mutation in early-onset Alzheimer's disease. Lancet 337:978

van Duijn CM, Van Broeckhoven C, Hardy JA, Goate AM, Rossor MN, Vandenberghe A, Martin JJ, Hofman A, Mullan MJ (1991c) Evidence for allelic heterogeneity in familial early onset Alzheimer's disease. Brit J Psych 158:471–474

Yoshioka K, Miki T, Katsuya T, Ogihara T, Sakaki Y (1991) The ^{717}Val→Ile substitution in amyloid precursor protein is associated with familial Alzheimer's disease regardless of ethnic groups. Biochem Biophys Res Commun 178:1141–1146

Locus Heterogeneity of Alzheimer's Disease

A. Roses, M. Pericak-Vance, M. Alberts, A. Saunders, H. Taylor,
J. Gilbert, C. Schwartzbach, M. Peacock, J. Fink, R. Bhasin,
and *D. Goldgaber*

Alzheimer's disease is heterogeneous: more than a single genetic mutation
accounts for several of the early onset AD recognizable phenotypes, and more
than one genetic locus is linked to late onset and early onset phenotypes.
Heterogeneity means different things to many investigators so it is important to
define clearly the terms of reference. Locus heterogeneity may mean that AD
is several totally independent processes that eventually develop into the clinical
and pathologic picture defined as AD. However, it may also refer to several
different loci involved in a common pathogenesis. In that case it may be
possible to piece together the puzzle of disease pathogenesis by defining the
relevant gene loci that contribute to the phenotype (Table 1).

Genetic diseases are usually thought about as simple Mendelian traits which,
when mutated, lead to the production of a predictable phenotype. In fact, in
Mendelian disorders the identical clinical phenotype can result from multiple
mutations at different loci in the genome (McKusick, 1990). As an example,
mutations in different subunits of an enzyme can cause the same clinical
disorder. Thus, whether the name now applied to diseases of hexosaminidase
subunits is Tay-Sachs disease (Hex-A, CH 14q locus) or Sandhoff's Disease
(Hex-B, CH 5q), it is very clear that different loci producing different mutations in subunits of the same enzyme can result in an identical clinical picture.
The subtypes can be differentiated only by testing for the precise mutation. If
these diseases were examined using linkage techniques, hetereogeneity at two
loci would be found, one on chromosome 15 and the other on chromosome 5.

Table 1. Locus Heterogeneity: Possible Mechanisms of Disease Expression

1. Subunits of the same enzyme or protein, coded at distinct loci
2. Interactive proteins, such as enzyme and substrate, e.g., APP (chromosome 21) and a
   serine protease (chromosome 19)
3. Expression-specific factors and polymorphic substances, e.g., neuronal cell type-specific
   factor and a specific form of constitutive protein
4. Two or more independently acting factors whose combined effects exceed individual
   expression, or can be increased by environment, e.g., Bombay blood type effect of blood
   transfusion (see text)
5. Age of onset lowered (rate of development increased) be independent mechanisms, e.g.,
   leakage of mutant APP with increased β-amyloid deposition slowly over an extended time
   period catalyzes an independent genetic (multiple determinant) process

F. Boller et al. (Eds.)
Heterogeneity of Alzheimer's Disease
© Springer-Verlag Berlin Heidelberg 1992

Table 2. Evidence for Locus Heterogeneity in Alzheimer's Disease

1. APP770^{717} mutations-chromosome 21q
   Three different base mutations at the same codon
2. Chromosome 19q linkage of late onset familial AD
3. Several large, unlinked early onset familial AD families, including the Volga-German group (excluded from chromosome 21 and chromosome 19)
4. Status of two large early onset familial AD families (FAD4 and AD/A) that exclude the APP locus, but show possible centromeric chromosome 21 linkage

The controversies concerning whether or not Alzheimer's disease(s) is (are) genetic are primarily based on the difficulty of recognizing a major genetic (Mendelian) component in the older population. As more families have been identified and studied carefully, a sub-group of "genetic" AD families has been defined by linkage strategies. What proportion of AD is genetic is currently defined practically by what proportion can be recognized in the population as the direct result of a major Mendelian trait producing recognizable "genetic" families. Another viewpoint looks at the AD phenotype as the result of multiple, interacting genetic loci and provides major research opportunities. A mutation at certain loci may be sufficient to result in a recognizable autosomal dominant inherited phenotype (see below, APP717 mutations in early-onset AD). Other mutations may be interactive, conferring susceptibility when two, three, or more loci provide interactive polymorphic traits. There are many well-documented, multi-locus interactions that lead to the expression of genetic traits. Such a relationship is called epistasis by geneticists (Ott, 1991). The contribution of several genetic loci to the expression of a complex disease phenotype can be used constructively to search for relevant genes.

Locus heterogeneity is supported by the currently available data in AD (Table 2; St. George-Hyslop et al., this volume). Multiple loci must be differentiated from the heterogeneity that can occur at a single locus. The viewpoint of many prominent AD investigators is that abnormalities of the amyloid precursor protein gene (APP, coded at a locus on CH21q13.3) or direct, pathogenic effects of the APP gene product define the mechanism for the development of AD (Beyreuther and Masters, 1991; Selkoe, 1990; Koh et al., 1990; Yankner and Mesulam, 1991; Younkin, 1991). The recent delineation of three different mutations of APP leading to early AD provided support to the champions of central APP dogma (Goate et al., 1991; Murrel et al., 1991; Chartier-Harlin et al., 1991). However, careful and exhaustive sequencing of APP exon 17 (where all three mutations were described at codon 717), and of the entire APP cDNA, have yet to delineate other mutations associated with AD. Mutations of APP have been associated with other syndromes (Levy et al., 1990; see also Fig. 1). The first identifed APP 770$^{\text{Ile}717}$ mutation was described in two large families. In both families there was *prior positive genetic evidence for a CH21 locus and no recombination between the APP gene and AD* (Goate et al., 1989; Pericak-Vance et al., 1988). Subsequent families were found by screening all available families and many "sporadic" cases (Hardy et al., 1991; Naruse et al., 1991). "Sporadic" cases automatically became "genet-

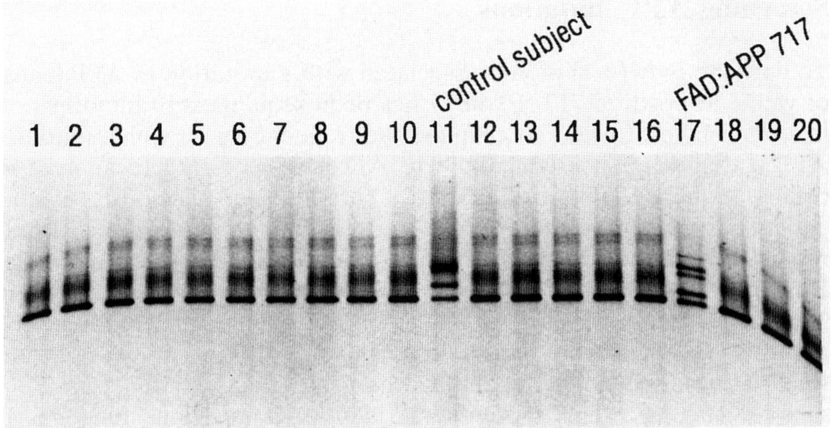

Fig. 1. Denaturing gradient gel electrophoresis of APP cDNA (exons 14 through 17). mRNA was extracted from postmortem cerebellum samples of control subjects and patients with AD. Following reverse transcription, APP cDNA was amplified as a series of overlapping fragments, each of which was analyzed by denaturing gradient gel electrophoresis. DGGE analysis of APP cDNA fragments representing exons 14 through 17 is shown. Lane 17 contains material from a patient with familial AD known to have the APP717^{IIe} mutation. Lane 11 contains material from a control subject and displays a unique DGGE polymorphism. This indicates that this subject is heterozygous for a novel point mutation in this region of APP. The single homoduplex bands in the remaining lanes indicates that these samples are homozygous throughout this region of the APP coding sequence

ic" as soon as the mutation was found. Perhaps this result might contribute to the acceptance of the fact that "sporadic" is a term that reflects our ignorance and that, as more AD genes are defined, this unknown category of AD will diminish. The fact that the APP locus has been excluded by recombination events in virtually all other large early onset and late onset families is sometimes ignored. In fact, APP may well play a central role in the pathogenesis of the AD phenotype without having to place a mutation in the gene itself. Expressed genes, coded elsewhere in the genome, may interact with APP or β-amyloid to produce the disease. Therefore, a genetic linkage strategy based on defining possible epistatic relationships could lead directly to the discovery of currently unrecognized, relevant interacting genes (Table 2).

Several papers have recently reported transgenic transmission using APP gene constructs (Wirak et al., 1991; Quon et al., 1991; Kawabata et al., 1991). The most exciting paper reported the development of neuropathological findings including plaques, tangles, and cell loss identical to human AD in the transgenic mice (Kawabata et al., 1991). This supported the widely accepted view that a primary effect of APP was causative to the entire range of AD neuropathology, not simply increased amyloid production when the gene is overexpressed. Unfortunately, this paper has been retracted amidst an ongoing investigation by the National Institutes of Health, and any conclusions derived from this well-publicized paper should also be withdrawn.

Screening APP mutations

To date the *only* form of AD associated with a mutation in APP leads to a loss of valine at position 717. Exon 17 has been sequenced in hundreds of patients in several laboratories. To estimate the frequency with which mutations in the APP coding sequence contribute to AD it is necessary to analyze the entire coding sequence, not just exon 17. Hundreds of rigorously diagnosed AD patients must be analyzed. To be certain that polymorphisms do not simply represent sequence variants, samples from hundreds of controls must also be analyzed. Unfortunately, the relatively high error rate of automated DNA sequencing precludes its use in this context. Denaturing gradient gel electrophoresis (DGGE) is an extremely sensitive method to detect point mutations, small inserts, and deletions and can be used effectively for a large number of samples (Fig. 1). This method has identified mutations in genes for many disorders, including hemophilia, thalassemia, cystic fibrosis, retinitis pigmentosa, Albright's hereditary osteodystrophy, phenylketonuria, Lesch-Nyhan syndrome, and familial Creutzfeldt-Jakob disease. Using DGGE, DNA fragments are electrophoresed through an increasing gradient of chemical denaturant. DNA fragments stop migrating when they reach a concentration of denaturant that causes them to partially melt. Since point mutations alter the tendency to melt, DNA amplified from alleles differing by a single nucleotide can be resolved as two homoduplex bands. Furthermore, heating and reannealing amplification products create heteroduplexes (DNA strands arising from alleles which differ by a single nucleotide), which further confirms that the sample is heterozygous for a point mutation.

Figure 1 illustrates the utility of DGGE in selecting samples for direct DNA sequence analysis using amplified exons 14–17 of APP cDNA from 20 different postmortem brain samples. Two samples were clearly different: #11 was from a Rapid Autopsy Protocol disease control and #17 from an autopsy on a patient with the APP770$^{\mathrm{Ile}717}$ mutation. This control sample was further characterized (J. K. Fink and M. L. Peacock) and was found to contain a point mutation in the β-amyloid coding sequence, in exon 16. There was no evidence of AD on neuropathological examination. The clear difference between DGGE polymorphisms in lanes #11 and #17 indicates that the point mutations are not the same. The single homoduplex bands in the remaining samples indicate that those samples are homozygous throughout this region of the APP coding sequence.

Thus there are now mutations of APP at or near the β-amyloid coding sequence that are *not* associated with early onset AD. While this does not change the support for an APP770^{717} mutation causing a rare form of early onset AD, it further isolates this specific site of mutation as the only known causative, direct link between APP and AD. Thus tissues from individuals with one of the APP770^{717} mutations have become most relevant for studying pathogenesis. Studying the mechanism through which this specific mutated gene product interacts with other genes or gene products to cause AD may well provide a context for identifying other relevant factors.

Summary of the current genetic data

Early-onset Alzheimer's disease
(mean age of onset in families before age 60)

The first paper reporting linkage in AD families described positive lod scores in a multipoint analysis using chromosome 21 probes in four early onset familial AD families with apparent autosomal dominant inheritance (St George-Hyslop et al., 1987). A careful review of that paper demonstrates that the largest proportion of positive data came from one family, designated FAD4. The following year Schellenberg et al. (1988) excluded chromosome 21 linkage in an independent series of early onset AD families as well as in a set of Volga-German origin pedigrees. In a paper excluding chromosome 21 linkage in a series of late onset AD pedigrees, Pericak-Vance et al. (1988) pointed out a single early onset AD pedigree (DUK372) in their series in which there was the maximum possible positive lod score with chromosome 21 probes, representing the only positive chromosome 21 data in the series. Goate et al. (1989) then reported positive chromosome 21 data in six families, but again virtually all the data came from one large early onset AD family, designated family #21. Selection of chromosome 21-positive families from the various series allowed a respectable lod score to be added together, but defied a scientific rationale for selection. Recombination events were documented between the disease locus and the APP gene probes in all four of the original St George-Hyslop et al. (1987) families, but no cross-overs were found in family 21 or DUK372. Goate et al. (1991) used primers that had detected an APP770^{683} mutation in heredi-tary cerebral hemorrhage with amyloidosis of the Dutch type (Levy et al., 1990), and detected a mutation in codon 717 (APP770^{Ile717}) that predicted a valine to phenylalanine change in affected members of family 21 and DUK 372. No families with the APP 770^{717} mutation were found by Schellenberg et al. (1992). Subsequently a few small families in Japan and France were found to have this mutation (Naruse et al., 1991; Hardy et al., 1991). St George-Hyslop et al. report a Canadian family of British descent in this volume. A large Indiana family that was not part of any previously published linkage series demonstrated a second mutation at codon 717 (Murrel et al., 1991). Chartier-Harlin et al. (1991) then found another small British family with a third mutation at codon 717. Thus the first genetic lesion causing early onset AD involves the loss of a valine (to isoleucine, glutamine, or glycine). The mechanism or process "causing" AD remains unknown (see below, Interaction of APP with other candidate genes).

The status of chromosome 21 linkage in the remaining large early onset families is still unclear. One family in the original St George-Hyslop et al. series, FAD4, continues to be linked to several probes on the centromeric side of APP (Tanzi et al., 1991). In FAD4, APP is excluded as the gene by several recombination events. Even so, the APP cDNA was completely sequenced in this family and no mutation was found (Tanzi et al., 1991). Pulst et al. (1991) have excluded linkage to the pericentromeric region of chromosome 21 in another of the original St George-Hyslop et al. (1987) families, FAD1. The residual data for linkage to chromosome 21 probes in all but one other published family are less compelling or frankly negative. In fact, there remain very little data, other than FAD4 and another large family reported by van Broeckhoven et al. (1987), to support another locus on chromosome 21 once the codon 717 mutation family data are subtracted.

Late-onset familial Alzheimer's disease (mean age of onset in families > 60 years)

Pericak-Vance et al. (1991) reported chromosome 19 linkage in a series of primarily late onset AD families. They used the Affected Pedigree Member analysis (Weeks and Lange, 1988) as a screening method and then confirmed the Affected Pedigree Member association data by standard likelihood (lod score method) analyses using several chromosome 19 probes. Since the mean age of onset in their series was close to 70 years of age, obvious autosomal dominant inheritance was far less likely to be apparent. Yet by linking these families to chromosome 19, the existence of a genetic factor was supported. Schellenberg and his collaborators studied an independent series of late onset AD families and reported positive lod scores (over 2.0) with three highly polymorphic, microsatellite chromosome 19q probes (Ropers et al., 1992; Schellenberg et al., 1992). Mullan and his collaborators also analyzed a third small series of late onset families using the Affected Pedigree Member method and found statistical significant association to chromosome 19 probes (Ropers et al., 1992). Thus, these now is general support for chromosome 19q linkage in late onset AD.

The recent consensus of linkage of chromosome 19 introduces a distinct change in the prevailing opinions concerning the genetics of AD. The APP770^{717} mutations have confirmed the view of the dedicated amyloidologists, at least in one, uncommon early onset form of the disease. The emerging data for late onset familial AD linkage on chromosome 19 strengthens the rationale for using a genetic approach focusing on 19q. The remaining subsets of apparently early onset familial AD families that exhibit Mendelian inheritance remain unlinked and provide a strong rationale for continuing genetic linkage screening of the genome. The other genes that contribute to linkage, other than APP, may be related to APP, or may be part of a distinct mechanism. As described below, a hypothesis that favors gene product interactions can be very helpful in selecting candidate genes from linked regions for further testing.

Two-locus modelling

Although the conventional view of genetic diseases is usually that of a single Mendelian trait sufficient to produce disease in either one dose (autosomal dominant) or two doses (autosomal recessive), multifactorial diseases are well described (Ott, 1991). The expression of genetic traits due to the interactions of two loci is common. When the trait is morbidly recognized as a disease, the term used is multigenic. Whether the result is the expression of a trait such as a blood type, or the fatal reaction of individuals expressing that trait to a blood transfusion, the genetic basis is known and accepted. Late onset AD may be the expression of interacting traits to produce disease.

A multigenic trait may produce morbid consequences by interaction with environmental factors. The Bombay blood type results from the interaction of a particular enzyme on the glycoprotein responsible for the ABO blood type. This multiprotein interaction has no health consequences unless these individuals receive a blood transfusion. Because they make antibodies to A, B and O blood types, any transfusion can be fatal. Thus, the action of a genetically specified enzyme on a genetically specified glycoprotein substrate produces either no symptoms or a potentially fatal disease, depending on the environment. This genetic trait can be detected by a biochemical test. If families expressing this trait were tested for linkage, the genetic loci of both the enzyme and the substrate would be detected using a two-locus model.

If, in fact, late onset AD is a multigenic disease, linkage data would define the chromosomal loci even without a direct biochemical test. Published data already illustrate several interesting peculiarities that suggest multigenic factors in AD. Analysis of late onset AD families using the Affected Pedigree Member method supports an association to both chromosome 19 and chromosome 21 loci (Pericak-Vance et al., 1991). When the lod score method of analysis is used, the chromosome 21 locus is excluded but chromosome 19 lod scores are positive. Yet the chromosome 19 lod scores are maximally positive when affected members-only are used in the lod score analyses. The usual age curve lod score analyses generally contribute additional data to lod scores, but are less positive in late onset AD. However, preliminary analyses combining chromosome 19 and chromosome 21 loci in a two-locus model increase the age curve lod scores (Haines et al., 1992). Thus, there are intriguing preliminary suggestions that loci on chromosomes 21 and 19 may interact to contribute to the late onset AD phenotype. This type of analysis may prove increasingly valuable in testing informative loci at or near candidate genes.

Interaction of APP with other candidate genes

The genetic analyses of mutations at APP codon 717 (of 770) support the notion that these mutations, leading to an amino acid substitution for a valine, are sufficient but not necessary for the development of early onset AD. The mechanism of disease production and the role of mutated APP in these individuals are still unknown. Although these may be quite distinct, it is not known how and where amyloid protein is formed from its precursor. APP is a transmembrane glycoprotein with the β-amyloid region located close to the carboxy-terminal end of the precursor. There are two events that normally prevent formation of amyloid. First, APP spans the membrane in such a way that the carboxy-terminous of the β-amyloid region is buried within the membrane and, therefore, is not available for the proteolytic cleavage that is required to generate the β-amyloid fragment. Second, normal maturation of the secreted

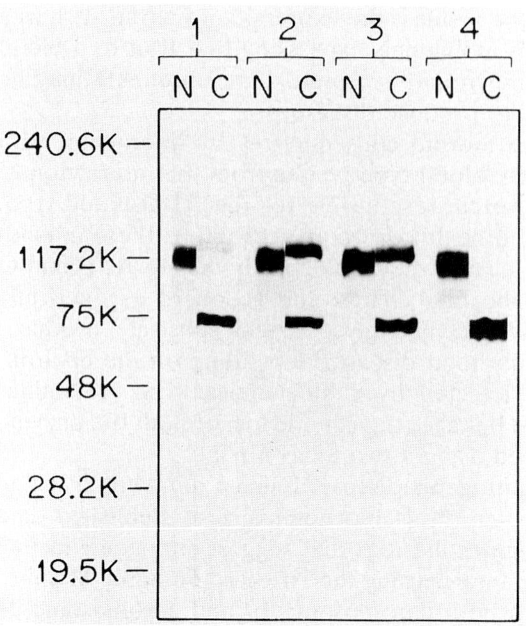

Fig. 2. Western blot of extracellular APP in media from recombinant baculovirus-infected cells. Four samples were prepared from the media of four recombinant baculovirus-infected cells:
#1 APP751
#2 APP751 with val to IIe mutation at codon 717 of the APP770 form
#3 APP751 with glu to gln mutation at codon 683 of the APP770 form
#4 APP751 with most of β-amyloid and C-terminal deleted.
Media were harvested, clarified by centrifugation and ultracentrifugation, concentrated and electrophesed. After Western blotting each lane was cut lengthwise into two parts. Each half was stained with antibodies directed to the N-terminal (N) and C-terminal (C) of APP. Note that the N-terminal antibody recognized approximately equal amounts of total secreted APP in all three samples. Surprisingly, the C-terminal antibody detected APP in all three samples, but not in control truncated APP that does not have the C-terminus. The amount of C-terminus containing APP is increased in samples of APP from either the early onset AD mutation (lane 2) or the Hereditary Cerebral Hemorrhage with Amyloidosis – Dutch type mutation (lane 3). [Bhasin and Goldgaber]

form of the precursor effectively precludes formation of β-amyloid because its involves cleavage within the β-amyloid region. Goldgaber and colleagues have produced recombinant APP with and without mutations. They used the baculovirus expression system to demonstrate proteolytic cleavage at the proper site. The baculovirus expression system produces cells with a very high proportion of their protein content as APP. They also detected small amounts of secreted APP molecules that were not proteolytically processed and contained amino- and carboxy-terminus of the holoprotein. Increased numbers of secreted but uncut APP are present in the extracellular media with either the AD Val717-IIe or the Hereditary Cerebral Hemorrhage with Amyloidosis-Dutch type Glu683-Gln mutations. Western blots of extracelluar media were examined with N-terminal and C-terminal antibodies to APP. Unprocessed APP appears extracellularly in increased amounts, without constitutive proteolytic cleavage when the mutant constructs are used (Fig. 2).

We established fibroblast cultures from AD patients and relatives from DUK 372 (Fig. 3). Analysis of APP found in the media of fibroblast cell lines from two patients revealed the presence of APP with carboxy-terminus. Quantitative comparisons with fibroblast cultures from other affected and clinically unaf-

Fig. 3. Western blot of extracellular APP in media from cultured human fibroblasts. Media from skin fibroblasts from two patients with the APP770$^{\text{Ile717}}$ mutation were harvested, clarified by centrifugation including. 100,000 xg for 1 hour at 4°C, and partially purified and concentrated. Following electrophoresis and Western blotting, each strip was divided into two halves longitudinally, and one half was stained with N-terminal antibodies to APP while the other half was stained with C-terminal antibodies. The strips were then mounted side by side. Both strips of both lanes show the presence of N-terminal (N) and C-terminal (C) containing APP of the same full length. [Bhasin and Goldgaber]

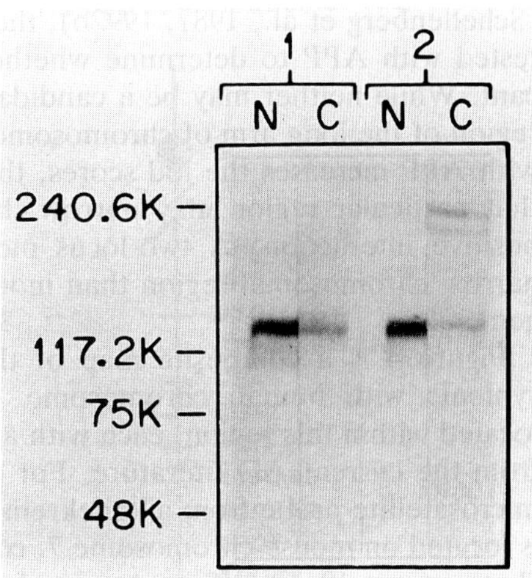

fected family members (with and without codon 717IIe mutation) are now in progress.

These data suggest that some APP could be released into the extracellular space without being proteolytically cut within the β-amyloid region. Thus, APP would be outside the membrane with both ends of the β-amyloid region available for proteolytic processing. A second point is that the mutations result in increased amounts of C-terminus containing APP secreted into the extracellular space. Specific mutations seem to interfere with efficient retention of APP in the membrane. Where proteolytic processing of these APP molecules would take place is not known. It could be taking place in the extracellular space or APP could be taken in by scavenger cells like microglia and degraded into amyloid, and then excreted into the extracellular space. Thus, in the only example where APP is known to cause an early onset AD, the loss of a valine at codon 717 leads to a transposition to the extracellular space of unprocessed APP. These data are clearly relevant to the large number of studies concentrating on the intracellular metabolism of APP. A similar mechanism may account for the vascular distribution of β-amyloid in Hereditary Cerebral Hemorrhage with Amyloid-Dutch type.

Other early onset AD pedigrees clearly exclude the APP locus as the major gene. Other loci may eventually be found to be sufficient to produce the AD phenotype in these families. Genomic screening continues in these families as a research priority. Late onset AD is currently being tested using two-locus modelling with several chromosome 19 loci and APP.

It is useful to illustrate how the APP locus on chromosome 21 is used in combination with other loci for early or late onset AD. A highly polymorphic microsatellite polymorphism, gt12, is located very close to the APP gene. This genetic marker is not linked to late onset AD using the lod score method. Yet it is possible to use gt12 in combination with other genetic markers in a two-locus model. Since positive lod scores are obtained with ATP1A3 and KLK1

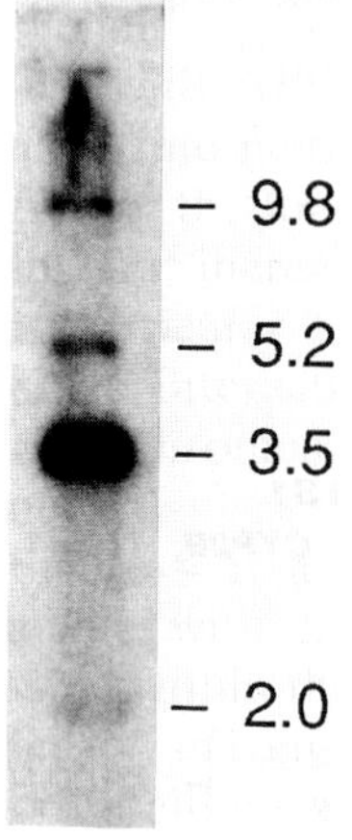

Fig. 5. Chromosome 19 cosmid clone hybrized with APP770. DNA from the insert of a human cosmid clone, designated D10, was cut with Pst1 and electrophoresed on a 1% agarose gel. This figure is an autoradiograph (Southern blot) hybridized with radiolabelled APP 770, then washed with moderate stringency conditions. Several positive hybridization bands are illustrated. The darkest band is approximately 3.6 kb, with clear bands at 2, 5.2, and 9.8 kb. This cosmid clone was identified from chromosome 19 cosmid panels provided by Dr. Pieter deJong of the Lawrence Livermore National Laboratory and has been mapped to 19q13.1. Similar data have been obtained from other independently generated chromosome 19-specific genomic clones (see text)

coded on chromosome 19, are part of a more detailed manuscript (Alberts and Roses, manuscript in preparation). The finding of amyloid-like genes in chromosome 19 may help to clarify the role of the proteins that form amyloid and amyloid plaques in the pathogenesis of AD.

As additional examples of mapping strategies starting with highly polymorphic probes without a pathogenetic rationale, positive lod scores exist for CEA and ATP1A3. Both have informative microsatellite markers located close to each other on 19q13.2. This region is genetically quite distinct from the region of the kallekrein genes (19q13.4), but may be sufficiently close to be detected by current linkage analyses. Comparisons of the two 19q regions within the context of a two-locus genetic model may help define the location of a gene that interacts positively with APP to produce the phenotype of late onset AD. Of course it is also quite possible that APP is not the critical chromosome 21 locus to evaluate, and other loci can be used as well. Thus, an experimental framework exists to define the chromosomal regions contributing to the development of the AD phenotype, quite independent of any particular belief systems concerning the primacy of the APP gene in the development of AD. Two-locus modelling analyses are currently in progress in the laboratories of Drs. J. Haines (Massachusetts General Hospital) and M. Pericak-Vance (Duke University).

How much of Alzheimer's Disease is genetic?

It is not yet possible to answer this question accurately. It is important to point out that at least three varieties of one form of mutation, APP770[717], have been shown to be genetic during the past year. Although the detection of the mutation was precipitated by the presence of two large families with no recombinants with chromosome 21 probes adjacent to APP, all of the other small families were defined while searching for the mutation. Thus, there are obviously more genetic forms of AD than were known to exist in 1990. As discussed above, there are several well-studied early onset pedigrees with convincing genetic structure that remain unlinked. Late onset AD pedigrees have been linked to chromosome 19 genetic markers. As the data continue to develop, it is reasonable to point out that the presence of "non-genetic" cases within families that are being studied would tend to diminish the positive data for linkage. The effects of missed diagnoses, phenocopies, or other genetic forms of AD within studied pedigrees would work against finding positive linkage data. It is equally clear that, as research continues, more genetic mutations will be defined and, as a result, the proportion of "genetic" AD will increase.

In the chapter in this volume by St George-Hyslop et al., the authors raise "the possibility that the $APP770^{717}$ mutation per se may be more important in the timing of the onset of symptoms rather than being causative". This research group is collaborating with ours in studies of epistasis, so it is reasonable that they may have a similar viewpoint. They further state, "Obviously, the best evidence to support such a hypothesis would be the discovery of pedigrees in which the mutation is not present in all affected members, and the disease has a later age of onset in members without the mutation". DUK372 is just such a family. Figure 6 illustrates the extended pedigree of this family, which is one of the two reported by Goate et al. (1991). In the large sibship, all of the affected members have the $APP770^{717}$ mutation, with ages of onset of 53 (father, probably noticed later than others), 40, 49, 48, 51 and 51. Two of the other siblings below the age of 50 years have the mutation but have yet to develop diagnostic symptoms and signs of AD. Two living relatives, including a paternal cousin, have Probable Alzheimer's Disease with ages of onset at 65 and 68 years. Neither have the $APP770^{717}$ mutation, but both are included in linkage searches for other loci, including those on chromosome 19. With the discovery of the $APP770^{717}$ mutation we now have the opportunity to demonstrate heterogeneity within a pedigree. Whether an epistatic gene, "sporadic", or other descriptors are used as an explanation, the fact remains that the only distinguishing characteristic of the affected individuals is that their age of onset is more than a decade and a half later than other members of the family with the $APP770^{717}$ mutation.

Perhaps it is more reasonable to view each individual as a product of genetics and environment. Identical environments may produce an earlier disease in individuals with a particular susceptibility to an environmental factor. Multigenic diseases are rapidly being defined for illnesses of adult onset in which slow progression occurs throughout life. The definition of particular factors leading to the morbid expression of some of these diseases, such as atherosclerosis or AD, will no doubt allow the development of specific, rational therapies that interfere with some of the accelerating factors. As with other major advances in new discovery of the past decade (Koenig et al., 1987; Rommens et al., 1989; Riordan et al., 1989; Wallace et al., 1990; Viskochil et al., 1990), linkage analyses point our previously unknown relevant genes. The next challenge is how to design therapy making use of the relevant genetic information.

FAMILY   372

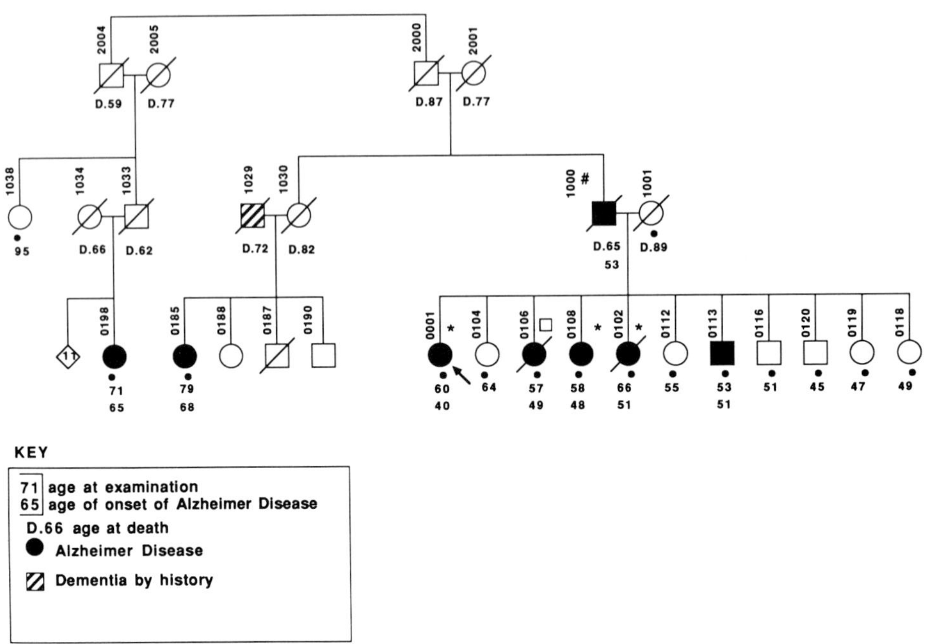

Fig. 6. Pedigree of North Carolina family with APP770^{Ile717} mutation. DNA from each individual designated with a dot was examined. In the five affected siblings with a mean age of onset of 49 years, each has the codon 717 Val-Ile mutation and an early onset AD. Several of the remaining clinically unaffected individuals also carry the mutation and are being followed prospectively. Individuals #0198 and 0185 have been diagnosed with probable AD, with onset at ages 65 and 68, respectively. These two individuals do not carry the mutation. Genotyping with other markers, involving highly polymorphic satellite probes from chromosome 19, demonstrate common genotypes. Thus the mutation may be superimposed on another gene(s), leading to earlier expression of disease

The operative question should not be how much of AD is genetic, but whether new discoveries in the genetics of AD can more rapidly lead to therapy in familial and sporadic AD. It is unfortunate that interim linkage results are not as descriptively satisfying or flashy as the latest attempts to test "accepted" hypotheses. In Duchenne muscular dystrophy, neurofibromatosis, cystic fibrosis, and most of the other genetic mutations identified using linkage strategies, the affected genes were totally unknown before discovery (DMD; Rommens et al., 1989; Riordan et al., 1989; Wallace et al., 1990; Viskochil et al., 1990). New discovery in AD will undoubtedly define the design of future rational and effective preventative therapies.

Acknowledgments. This work was supported by grants NS 19999 from the National Institutes of Health (A.D.R.), the Leadership in Excellence in Alzheimer's Disease Award (LEAD Award) AGO7922 from the NIA (A.D.R.),

M01-RR-30, National Center for Research Resources, General Clinical Research Centers Program, NIH, and research grants from the Alzheimer's Association (M.L.A., D.G.).

References

Alberts MJ, Pericak-Vance MA, Royal V, Bebout J, Gaskell PC, Thomas JT, Hung W-Y, Clark C, Earl N, Roses AD (1991) Genetic linkage analysis of nerve growth factor (beta) in familial Alzheimer's disease. Ann Neurol 30:216–219

Beyreuther K, Masters CL (1991) Amyloid precursor protein (APP) and ˜A4 amyloid in the etiology of Alzheimer's disease: precursor-product relationships in the derangement of neuronal function. Brain Pathol 1:241–251

Chartier-Harlin M-C, Crawford F, Houlden H, Warren A, Hughes D, Fidani L, Goate A, Rossor M, Roques P, Hardy J, Mullan M (1991) Early-onset Alzheimer's disease caused by mutations at codon 717 of the β-amyloid precursor protein gene. Nature 353:844–846

Goate A, Chartier-Harlin M-C, Mullan M, Brown J, Crawford F, Fidani L, Giuffra L, Haynes A, Irving N, James L, Mant R, Newton P, Rooke K, Roques P, Talbot C, Pericak-Vance MA, Roses AD, Williamson R, Rossor M, Owen M, Hardy J (1991) Segregation of a missense mutation in the amyloid precursor protein gene with familial Alzheimer's disease. Nature 349:704–706

Goate AM, Haynes AR, Owen MJ, Farrall M, James LA, Lai LY, Mullan MJ, Rossor MN, Haynes AR, Farrall M, Lai LYC, Roques P, Williamson R, Hardy JA (1989) Predisposing locus for Alzheimer's disease on chromosome 21. Lancet 1:352–355

Haines JL, St George-Hyslop PH, Rimmler JB, Yamaoka L, Kazantsev A, Tanzi RE, Gusella JF, Roses AD, Pericak-Vance MA (1992) Inheritance of multiple loci in familial Alzheimer's disease. Third International Conference of Alzheimer's Disease and Related Disorders, Abano Terme (Padova), Italy, July 12–17, 1992, in press

Hardy J, Mullan M, Chartier-Harlin M-C, Brown J, Goate A, Rossor M, Collinge J, Roberts G, Luthert P, Lantos P, Naruse S, Kaneko K, Tsuji S, Miyatake T, Shimizu T, Kojima T, Nakano I, Yoshioka K, Sakaki Y, Miki T, Kaysuya T, Ogihara T, Roses A, Pericak-Vance MA, Haan J, Roos R, Lucotte G, David F (1991) Molecular classification of Alzheimer's disease. Lancet 337:1342–1343

Kawabata S, Higgins GA, Gordon JW (1991) Amyloid plaques, neurofibrillary tangles and neuronal loss in brains of transgenic mice overexpressing a C-terminal fragment of human amyloid precursor protein. Nature 354:476–478

Koenig M, Hoffman EP, Bertelson CJ, Monaco AP, Feener C, Kunkel LM (1987) Complete cloning of the Duchenne muscular dystrophy (DMD) cDNA and preliminary genomic organization of the DMD gene in normal and affected individuals. Cell 50:509–517

Koh J, Yang LL, Cotman CW (1990) β-amyloid protein increases the vulnerability of cultured cortical neurons to excitotoxic damage. Brain Res 533:315–320

Levy E, Carman MD, Fernandez-Madrid IJ, Power MD, Lieberburg I, Van Duinen SG, Bots GTAM, Luyendijk W, Frangione B (1990) Mutation of the Alzheimer's disease amyloid gene in hereditary cerebral hemorrhage, Dutch type. Science 248:1124–1126

McKusick VA (1990) Mendelian inheritance in man. Catalogs of autosomal dominant, autosomal recessive, and X-linked phenotypes. Ninth edition. The Johns Hopkins University Press, Baltimore

Murrel J, Farlow M, Ghetti B, Benson MD (1991) A mutation in the amyloid precursor protein associated with hereditary Alzheimer's disease. Science 254:97–99

Naruse S, Igarashi S, Kobayashi H, Aoki K, Inuzuka T, Kaneko K, Shimizu T, Iihara K, Kojima T, Miyatake T, Tsuji S (1991) Mis-sense mutation Val-to-Ile in exon 17 of amyloid precursor protein gene in Japanese familial Alzheimer's disease. Lancet 337:978–979

Ott J (1991) Analysis of human genetic linkage. Revised edition. The Johns Hopkins Press, Baltimore

Pericak-Vance MA, Bebout JL, Gaskell PC Jr, Yamaoka LH, Hung W-Y, Alberts MJ, Walker AP, Bartlett RJ, Haynes CA, Welsh KA, Earl NL, Heyman A, Clark C, Roses AD (1991) Linkage studies in familial Alzheimer disease: Evidence for chromosome 19 linkage. Am J Human Genet 48:1034–1050

Pericak-Vance MA, Yamaoka LH, Haynes CS, Speer MC, Haines JL, Gaskell PC, Hung W-Y, Clark CM, Heyman AL, Trofatter JA, Eisenmenger JP, Gilbert JR, Lee JE, Alberts MJ, Dawson DV, Bartlett RJ, Earl NL, Siddique T, Vance JM, Conneally PM, Roses AD (1988) Genetic linkage studies in Alzheimer's disease families. Exp Neurol 102:271–279

Pulst S-M, Fain P, Cohn V, Nee LE, Polinsky RJ, Korenberg JR (1991) Exclusion of linkage to the pericentromeric region of chromosome 21 in the Canadian pedigree with familial Alzheimer's disease. Human Genet 87:159–161

Quon D, Wang Y, Catalano R, Scardina JM, Murakami K, Cordell B (1991) Formation of β-amyloid protein deposits in brains of transgenic mice. Nature 352:239–241

Riordan JR, Rommens JM, Kerem B-S, Alon N, Rozmahel R, Grzelczak Z, Zielenski J, Lok S, Plavsic N, Chou J-L, Drumm ML, Iannuzzi MC, Collins FS, Tsui L-C (1989) Identification of the cystic fibrosis gene: cloning and characterization of complementary DNA. Science 245:1066–1072

Rommens JM, Iannuzzi MC, Kerem B-S, Drumm ML, Melmer G, Dean M, Rozmahel R, Cole JL, Kennedy D, Hidaka N, Zsiga M, Buchwald M, Riordan JR, Tsui L-C, Collins FS (1989) Identification of the cystic fibrosis gene: chromosome walking and jumping. Science 245:1059–1065

Ropers HH, Pericak-Vance MA, Siciliano M, Mohrenweiser H (1992) Report on the 2nd International Workshop on Human Chromosome 19. Cytogenet Cell Genet, in press

Saunders AM, Seldin MF (1990) A molecular genetic linkage map of mouse chromosome 7. Genomics 8:525–535

Schellenberg GD, Boehnke M, Wijsman EM, Moore DK, Martin GM, Bird TD (1992a) Genetic association and linkage analysis of the apolipoprotein CII locus and familial Alzheimer's disease. Ann Neurol 31:223–227

Schellenberg GD et al (1992) Report on the Second International Workshop on Human Chromosome 19. Cytogenet Cell Genet, in press

Schellenberg GD, Bird TD, Wijsman EM, Moore DK, Boehnke M, Bryant EM, Lampe TH, Nochlin D, Sumi SM, Deeb SS, Beyreuther K, Martin GM (1988) Absence of linkage of chromosome 21q21 markers to familial Alzheimer's disease. Science 241:1507–1510

Selkoe DJ (1990) Amyloid β-protein deposition as a seminal pathogenetic event in Alzheimer's disease. In: Natvig JB, Forre O, Husby G, Husebekk A, Skogen B, Sletten K, Westermark P (eds) Amyloid and amyloidosis. Dordrecht: Kluwer Academic Publishers, pp 713–717

St George Hyslop PH, Tanzi RE, Polinsky RJ, Haines JL, Nee L, Watkins PC, Myers RH, Feldman RG, Pollen D, Drachmann D, Growdon J, Bruni A, Foncin J-F, Salmon D, Frommelt P, Amaducci L, Sorbi S, Piacentini S, Stewart GD, Hobbs WJ, Conneally PM, Gusella JF (1987) The genetic defect causing familial Alzheimer's disease maps on chromosome 21. Science 235:885–890

Tanzi RE, Romano D, McClatchey A, Haines JL, Gusella JF, St George-Hyslop PH (1991) Analysis of the APP gene in familial Alzheimer's disease. Am J Human Genet 49 (Suppl):420

van Broeckhoven C, Genthe RAM, Vandenberghe A, Hosthemke B, Backhovens H, Raeymaekers P, Van Hul W, Wehnert A, Gheuns J, Cras P, Bruyland M, Martin JJ, Salbaum M, Multhaup G, Masters CL, Beyreuther K, Gurling HMD, Mullan MJ, Holland A, Barton A, Irving N, Williamson R, Richards SJ, Hardy JA (1987) Failure of familial Alzheimer disease to segregate with the A4-amyloid gene in several European families. Nature 329:153–155

Viskochil D, Buchberg AM, Xu G, Cawthon RM, Stevens J, Wolff RK, Culver M, Carey JC, Copeland NG, Jenkins NA, White R, O'Connell P (1990) Deletions and a translocation interrupt a cloned gene at the neurofibromatosis type 1 locus. Cell 62:187–192

Wallace MR, Marchuk DA, Andersen LB, Letcher R, Odeh HM, Saulino AM, Foundation JW, Brereton A, Nicholson J, Mitchell AL, Brownstein BH, Collins FS (1990) Type 1 neurofibromatosis gene: Identification of a large transcript disrupted in three NF1 patients. Science 249:181–186

Weeks DE, Lange K (1988) The affected pedigree member method for linkage analysis. Am J Human Genet 42:315–326

Wirak DO, Bayney R, Ramabhadran TV, Fracasso RP, Hart JH, Hauer PE, Hsiau P, Pekar SK, Scangos GA, Trapp BD, Unterbeck AJ (1991) Deposits of amyloid β protein in the central nervous system of transgenic time. Science 253:323–325

Yankner BA, Mesulam M-M (1991) β-amyloid and the pathigenesis of Alzheimer's disease. New Engl J Med 325:1849–1857

Younkin SG (1991) Processing of the Alzheimer's disease βA4 amyloid protein precursor (APP). Brain Pathol 1:253–262

Familial Alzheimer's Disease in Germans from Russia: A Model of Genetic Heterogeneity in Alzheimer's Disease

T. D. Bird, E. M. Nemens, D. Nochlin, S. M. Sumi,
E. M. Wijsman, and *G. D. Schellenberg*

Summary

We have studied 28 kindreds with familial Alzheimer's disease (FAD) that are all descended from the ethnic group of Germans from Russia. Eighteen families were of Volga German ancestry, originating from the same two villages and containing 132 demented individuals. Mean age of onset in these 18 families was 61 years, and mean duration of disease to death was 9.5 yrs. The affected persons had clinically and neuropathologically typical Alzheimer's disease. Nineteen autopsies in eight families demonstrated classic amyloid neuritic plaques, neurofibrillary tangles and amyloid angiopathy. The plaques were β/A4 antibody positive and prion antibody negative. Ten families were of Black Sea German ancestry with 41 affected persons. Mean age of onset in this group was 71.4 years, significantly later than in the Volga German kindreds. There was autopsy documentation of AD in three Black Sea German families. The largest Volga German families showed no evidence of linkage to markers on chromosome 21 and revealed none of the known mutations in the amyloid precursor protein (APP) or PRIP (prion) genes. These families represent a model of genetic heterogeneity when compared with other reported FAD kindreds. Because of their common, isolated ethnic background, the Volga German families are likely to represent the founder effect and a single, as yet unidentified, autosomal dominant mutation. The Black Sea German kindreds may represent additional heterogeneity.

Introduction

In 1979, Cook and colleagues described three families with familial Alzheimer's disease (FAD). The families were assumed to be unrelated and their ethnic background was not mentioned. In 1988, we discovered that these three families and two additional FAD kindreds identified in our research program were all of Volga German ancestry and originated from the same two neighboring villages (Bird et al., 1988). We concluded that these families were likely to be related, to represent the genetic founder effect and to probably carry the same autosomal dominant mutation for AD. By 1989, we had identified two additional kindreds (Bird et al., 1989). Subsequently, we have systematically

F. Boller et al. (Eds.)
Heterogeneity of Alzheimer's Disease
© Springer-Verlag Berlin Heidelberg 1992

searched for further FAD pedigrees with this specific ethnic background, and the present report is a description of our results.

Historical background

The central region of what is now Germany was devastated by the Seven Years War in the 1750s. Soon thereafter, Catherine the Great, an ethnic German herself, became Tzarina of Russia. She recognized an urgent need to settle and farm the area along the Volga River in Southern Russia. In the 1760s she enticed several thousand poor German peasants to leave their homeland in Hessen and the Palatinate and migrate to the Volga region. Approximately 27,000 Germans undertook this trip between 1763 and 1766. They formed 104 original colonies or villages on both sides of the Volga. Specifically, the villages of Frank and Walter were founded on the Medvitz River, approximately 60 miles east of Saratov, by 500 and 400 German emigrants, respectively (Fig. 1). A second, later migration of approximately 42,000 Germans settled the Black Sea region around Odessa, primarily, between the years 1804 and 1810. This Black Sea group came from overlapping but additional regions of Germany and Prussia. These immigrants became successful farmers but strictly maintained their German identity and rarely mixed with the surrounding population. After several generations, land became scarce and the ethnic Germans were drafted into the Russian army. Between 1871 and 1914, more than 100,000 of these individuals emigrated to the mid-western and western states of the USA. It is the descendants of these persons who form the population for our study. The ethnic Germans remaining in the Soviet Union endured severe persecution during World War II and the Stalinist era, and vast numbers were relocated to Siberia and other distant regions of the country (Sallet, 1974; Koch, 1977; Scheuerman and Trafzer, 1985).

Methods

FAD families were ascertained through contacts with the local and national chapters of the American Historical Society of Germans from Russia and through newspaper requests in 20 western cities and towns known to have substantial populations of Germans from Russia (Bird, 1991). Probable FAD was defined as a kindred with at least three demented persons (with two exceptions in this study). Living affected family members were examined by one of the authors or by a local physician. We obtained all available medical records and death certificates (Bird et al., 1989). We interviewed spouses, siblings and children of demented individuals. Clinical criteria for probable AD were those suggested by McKhann and colleagues (1984), except that complete neurologic examinations and psychometric testing were not available for persons who died many years ago. Individuals were not considered demented unless the dementia was documented by records or confirmed by at least two separate family members. Age of onset was determined to be that age at which family members and records agreed that the individual first began showing

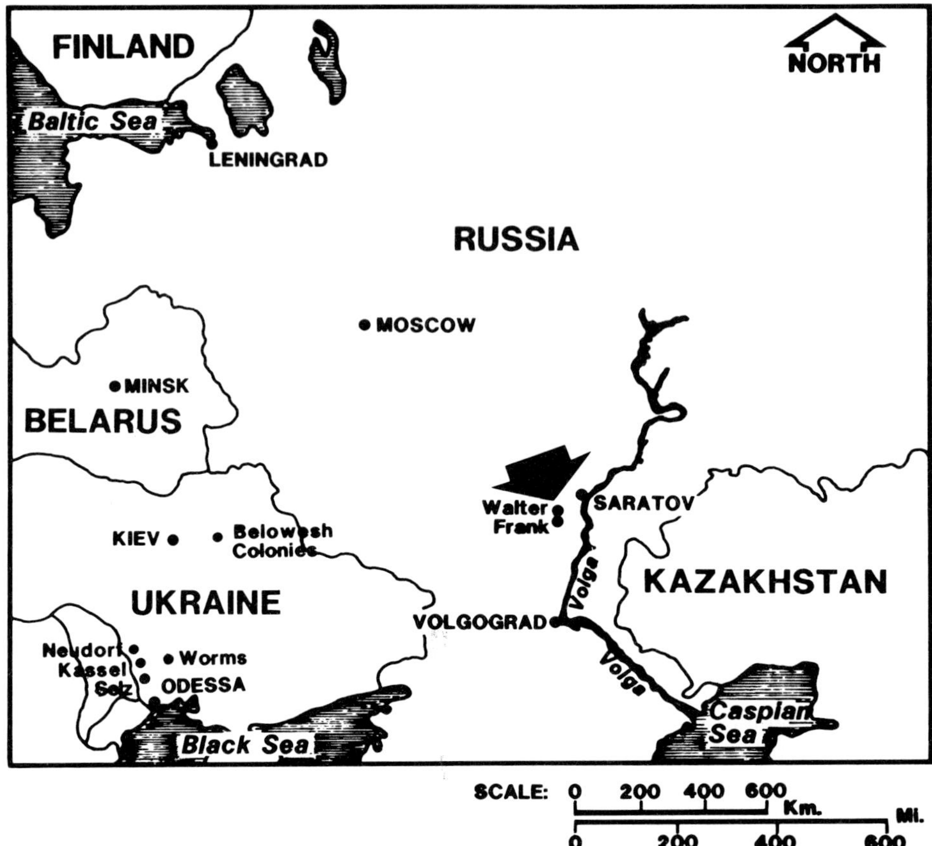

Fig. 1. Map of Russia and the Ukraine showing the villages of Frank and Walter on the Volga River and some of the Black Sea colonies

signs of memory loss or behavioral change. Mean age at onset, age at death and duration of disease were computed for each family. Comparisons between these means were performed using Student's t test. Linkage analysis was performed using previously described methods (Schellenberg et al., 1991b). We also obtained all detailed reports or actual specimens from autopsies. Twelve complete brain autopsies were performed at our institution and records or microscopic slides were reviewed from an additional 11 cases. We used the semiquantitative criteria for severity of AD adopted by CERAD (Bird et al., 1989; Mirra et al., 1991).

Volga German Kindreds

We ascertained 28 FAD kindreds of German/Russian background. Eighteen of these families were Volga German and all originated from the neighboring villages of Frank and Walter. The HB and KS pedigrees are illustrated in Figures 2 and 3. The 18 Volga German families contained 132 demented persons (65 males and 67 female). Two kindreds had 20 affected persons, two had 10–20 affected, 13 had three to nine affected and one had two affected. Mean age of onset was 61 years, mean age at death was 69 years and mean disease duration was 9.5 years (Table 1). Fourteen persons (11%) had an estimated onset at age 75 or older. These older individuals could represent coincidental sporadic "senile" AD or, alternatively, one end of the age of onset curve for the presumed AD gene. Mean age of onset in the males (59.1 years) was significantly earlier than in females (63.3 years, p < .01). Male and female mean ages at death were the same (68.8 and 69.3 years), but mean disease duration was longer in the males (10.1 vs 8.9 years, p < .05). This finding could represent an age of onset ascertainment bias in males, but the actual explanation is uncertain.

A review of 84 medical records in these 18 families revealed the following prevalence of clinical characteristics in addition to progressive dementia: language deficits (63%), rigidity or paratonia (31%), one or more seizures (19%), tremor (11%), and myoclonus (10%). These figures are obviously rough

Table 1. FAD in Germans from Russia: Kindreds Characteristics

	Volga Germans	p	Black Sea Germans	p
Numbers of families	18		10	
Number affected	132 (65 M, 67 F)		41 (21 M, 20 F)	
Age of onset (yrs)	61.09 ± 9.7		71.0 ± 7.6	.01
Range	40–84		57–89	
Males	59.1 ± 8.0	> .01	70.9 ± 9.0	> NS
Females	63.3 ± 10.6		71.9 ± 5.8	
Age at death (yrs)	69.0 ± 8.8		77.4 ± 7.6	.01
Range	50–90		71–93	
Males	68.8 ± 8.8	> NS	75.2 ± 6.7	
Females	69.3 ± 10		79.7 ± 5.8	
Disease duration (yrs)	9.5 ± 4.5		7.2 ± 3.1	.01
Range	3–23		1–12	
Males	10.1 ± 4.9	> .05	6.3 ± 3.6	> .01
Females	8.9 ± 4.0		8.5 ± 2.1	
Number of autopsies with AD	19		3	

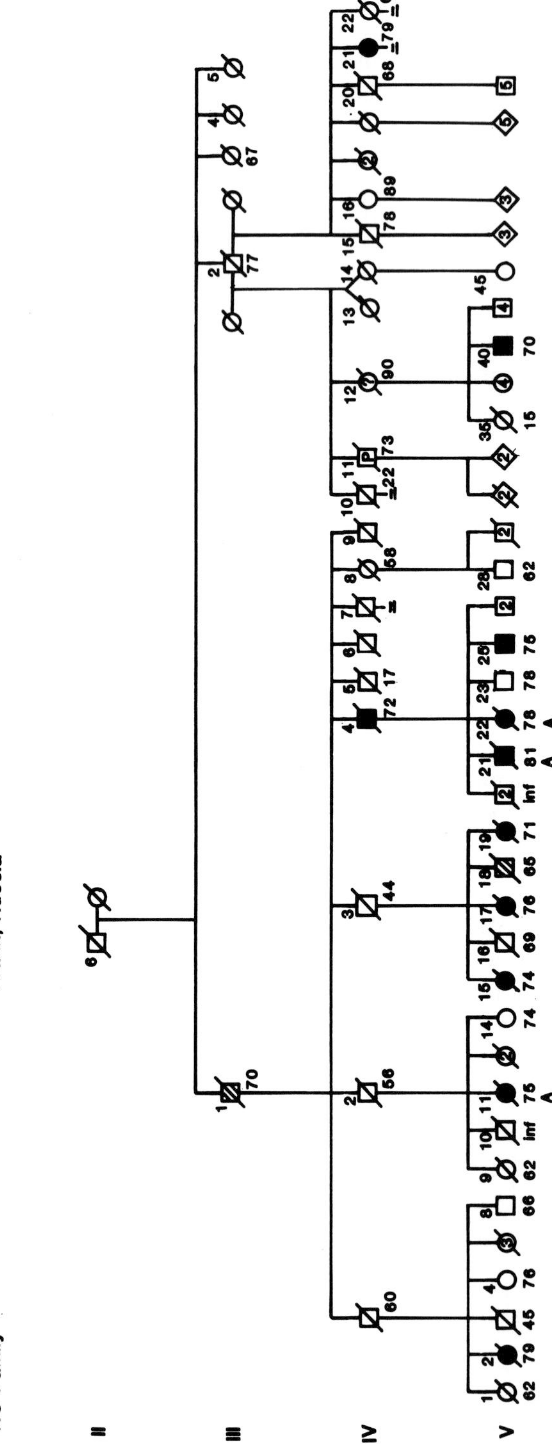

Fig. 2. The KS family from the Volga German village of Frank. Black symbols indicate dementia and cross-hatched symbols indicate probable dementia. Numbers under symbols are present ages or ages at death. Three autopsies (A) have confirmed AD

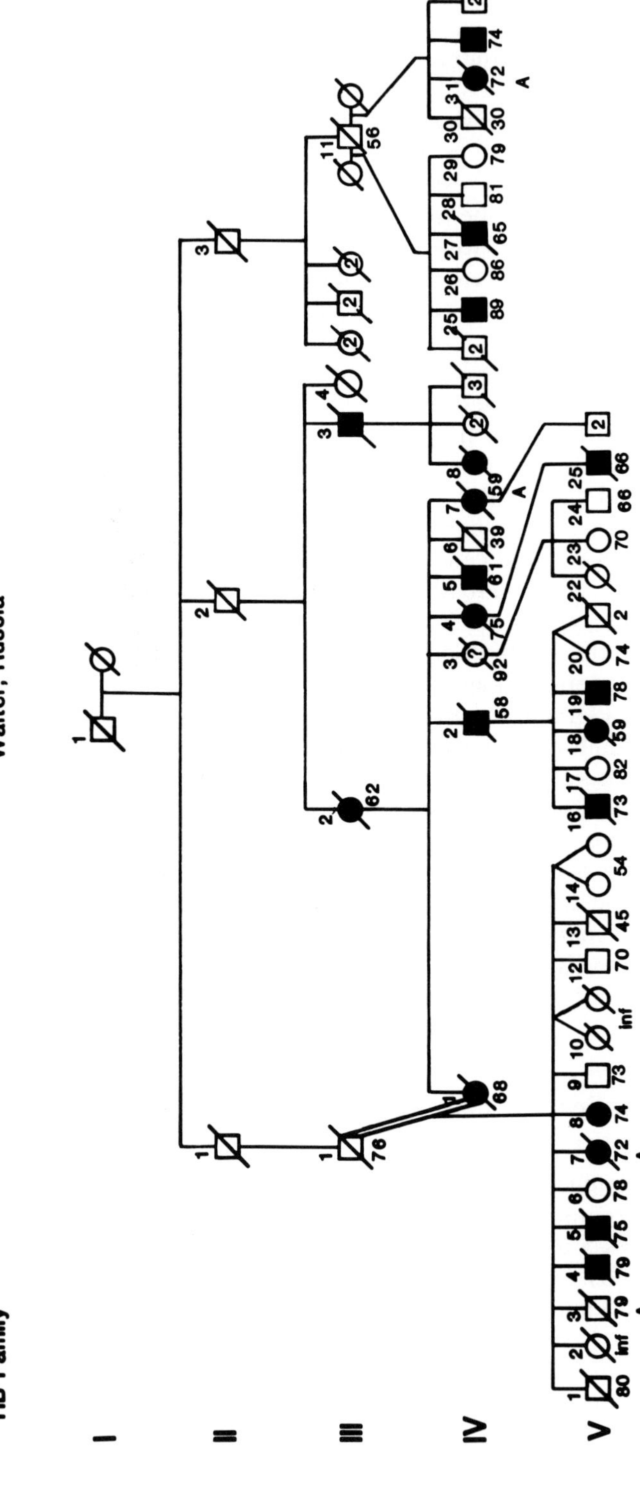

Fig. 3. The HB family from the Volga German village of Walter. Three autopsies (A) have confirmed AD. Symbols are the same as in Figure 2

approximations because many records never referred to the presence or absence of these clinical signs. We note that myoclonus and seizures are not uncommon in either sporadic or familial AD in the general population (Risse et al., 1990).

Several families share the same surname and we have been able to link three kindreds together in one instance and two others in another. However, no single common ancestor has been found for all families.

No fully documented instance of "non-penetrance" of the presumed AD gene was found. However, at least two persons with affected offspring survived past age 80 and were not recalled as being demented by other family members. These persons may represent lack of expression of the AD gene at advanced ages.

Nineteen autopsies were performed on demented persons in eight families. These autopsies showed the classic findings of AD, including neuritic amyloid plaques that were β/A4 antibody-positive and PRP antibody-negative, neurofibrillary tangles that were ALZ 50 antibody- and anti-tau antibody-positive, and amyloid angiopathy. Examples of the neuropathological findings are shown in Figure 4. One elderly patient (V-3) without clinical dementia from the HB family died from cancer, and examination of his brain showed only age-related changes. One individual in the E family had clinical and neuropathological changes typical of Creutzfeldt-Jakob disease, and is not included as a case of AD in this study (Cook et al., 1979; Bird et al., 1988).

A genetic linkage analysis (Table 2) was performed on the seven largest Volga German kindreds (Schellenberg et al., 1991b). The resulting lod scores were uniformly negative for all chromosome 21 markers, including D21S210, which is very tightly linked to the amyloid precursor protein (APP) locus, and D21S215, which is centromeric to D21S13. There were several obligate recombinations between affected members of these families and the APP region on chromosome 21. There were modestly positive but not significant lod scores with the Kell locus on chromosome 7 ($+ 1.26$, $\theta = .10$) and the CEA and D19S9 markers on chromosome 19 ($+ 1.52$, $\theta = .001$ and $+ 1.23$, $\theta = .15$, respectively). APP-717, APP-693 and known PRIP (prion) mutations were not found in DNA from these families (Schellenberg et al., 1991a).

Black Sea German Families

Ten families originated from villages in the Ukraine north of the Black Sea in the general vicinity of Odessa. The MMM and FZG pedigrees are shown in Figures 5 and 6. These families tended to be smaller than the Volga German kindreds, with fewer demented individuals. One family had two demented persons and the remainder had three to six affected individuals. There were 41 total affected persons (21 males and 20 females; Table 1). The mean age of onset of 71.4 years in the Black Sea kindreds was significantly later than the mean onset of 61 years in the Volga German families ($p < .01$). Mean age at death was also different between the two groups. In the Black Sea German

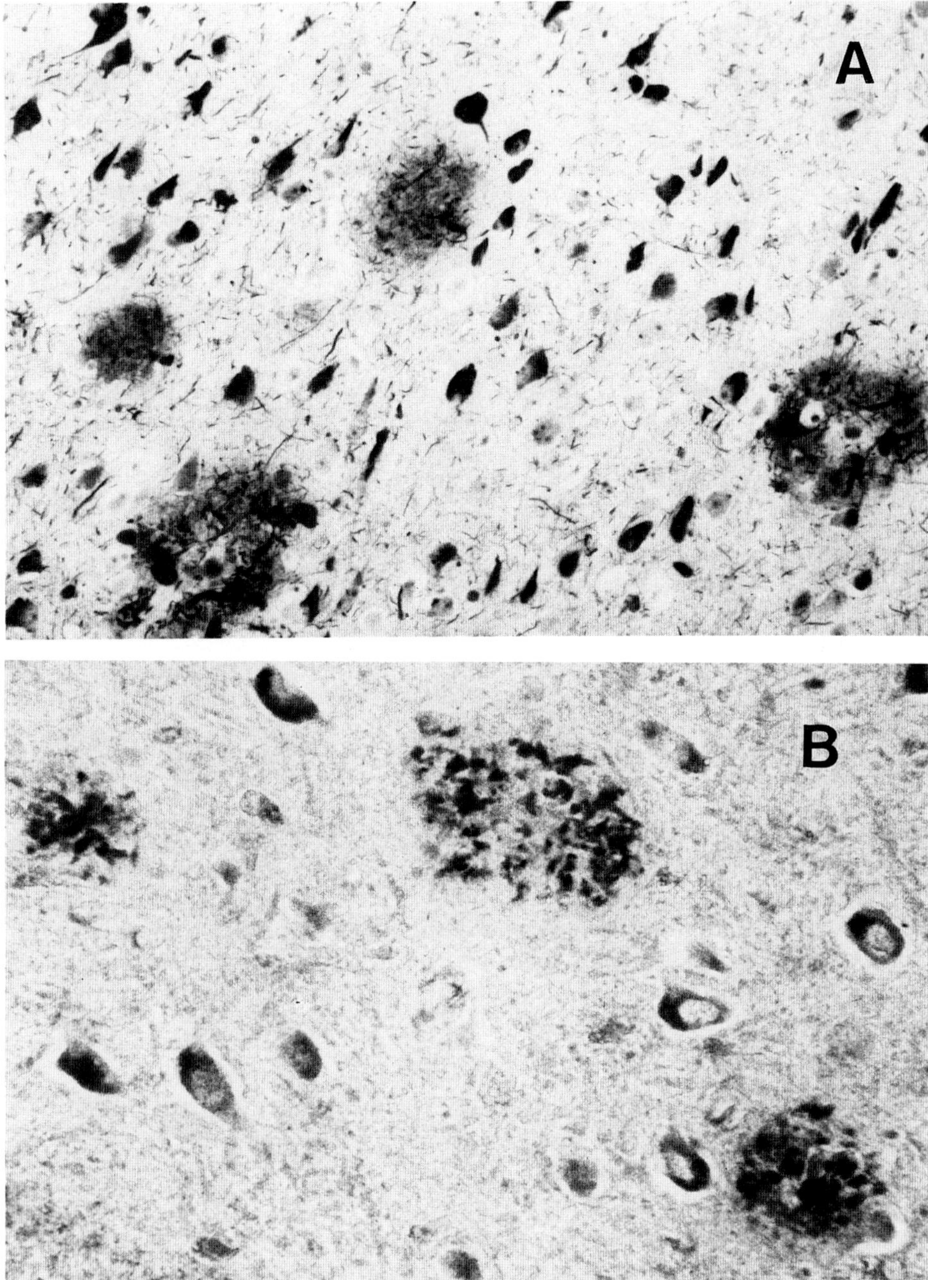

Fig. 4 A–C. Neuropathological micrographs showing: *A*) neuritic plaques and neurofibrillary tangles (Bielshowsky stain) from the hippocampus of M.W. in the Black Sea German/RR family; *B*) Amyloid plaques from the brain of IV-7 in the Volga German HB family, staining positive with an antibody to β/A4 amyloid (Masters and Beyreuther, polyclonal synthetic peptide to 1–42 aa sequence, 1:400); and *C*) cross-section of cerebral arterioles from R.W. in the Volga German W family, stained with β/A4 antibody

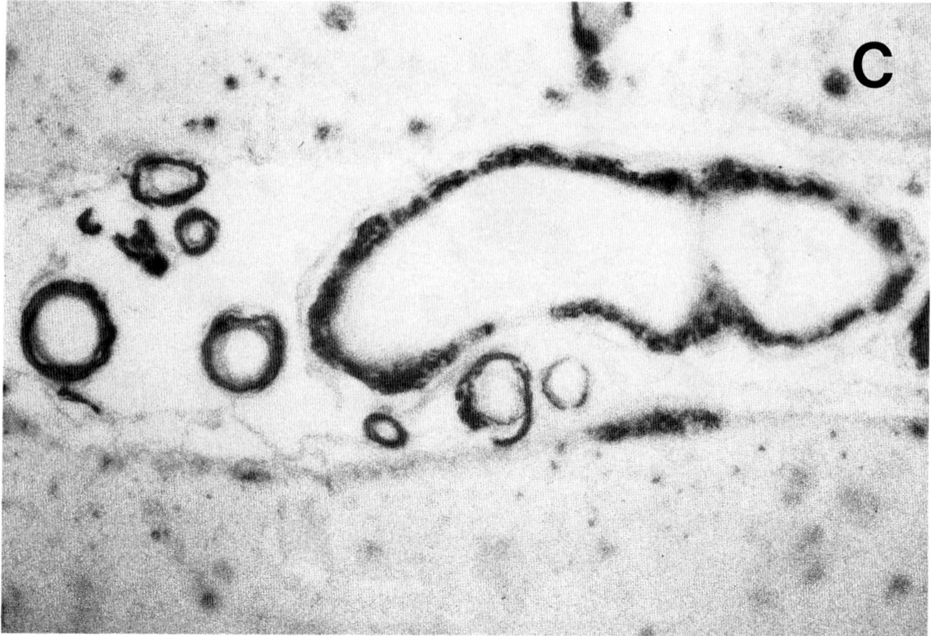

Fig. 4C

families, the males and females had a similar age of onset, but the mean disease duration was significantly shorter in the males (6.3 vs 8.5 years, respectively; p < .01). This latter finding may simply reflect an overall shorter longevity in the general population of males in their eighth decade of life relative to females. Mean disease duration was also shorter in the Black Sea males compared to the Volga German males, whereas there was no difference between the females. Two kindreds ascertained separately were later discovered to share a common blood relative.

Table 2. Chromosome 21 linkage Analysis: Volga German Kindreds*

Marker	Lod score	Recombination fraction (θ)
D21 S215	−2.20	.10
D21 S13/S16	−3.06	.10
D21 S1/S11	−4.06	.10
D21 S210	−2.64	.10
D21 S82	−3.76	.05
D21 S17	−1.96	.05
D21 S112	−2.55	.10
COL 6A1	−1.75	.05

* Analysis performed with q = .06 and age of onset correction

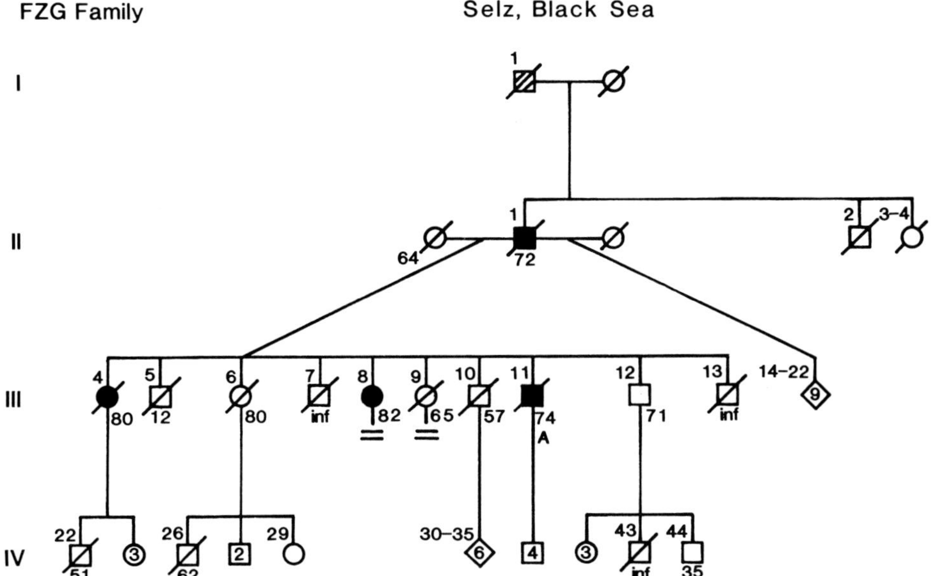

Fig. 5. The FZG family from the Black Sea village of Selz. Autopsy (A) confirmed AD in III-11. For symbols, see Figure 2

Conclusions

We draw the following conclusions from this study:

1. These kindreds represent clinically and neuropathologically typical Alzheimer's disease. The affected persons uniformly have the adult onset of a slowly progressive dementing disorder lasting approximately seven to ten years, associated with cerebral cortical atrophy, amyloid plaques, neurofibrillary tangles and amyloid angiopathy.

2. In most, if not all, of these families the disease presumably represents an autosomal dominant genetic disorder. Multiple generations are affected, males and females are equally affected and there is male-to-male transmission. Penetrance of the gene or genes is very high if individuals at risk survive into their 70s. There are only a few possible examples of lack of expression in elderly obligate gene carriers.

3. The genetic mutation is not likely to be in the APP gene or at any other location on chromosome 21. This makes these families different from recently reported kindreds with early onset FAD and proven point mutations in the APP gene (Goate et al., 1991). Therefore, these families are a model of genetic heterogeneity in FAD.

4. The Volga German kindreds are likely to represent the founder effect and to all carry the same FAD mutation. No common ancestor has been found and we have not yet traced the families back to the exact villages of origin in Germany. However, genetic homogeneity is likely in these 18 Volga Ger-

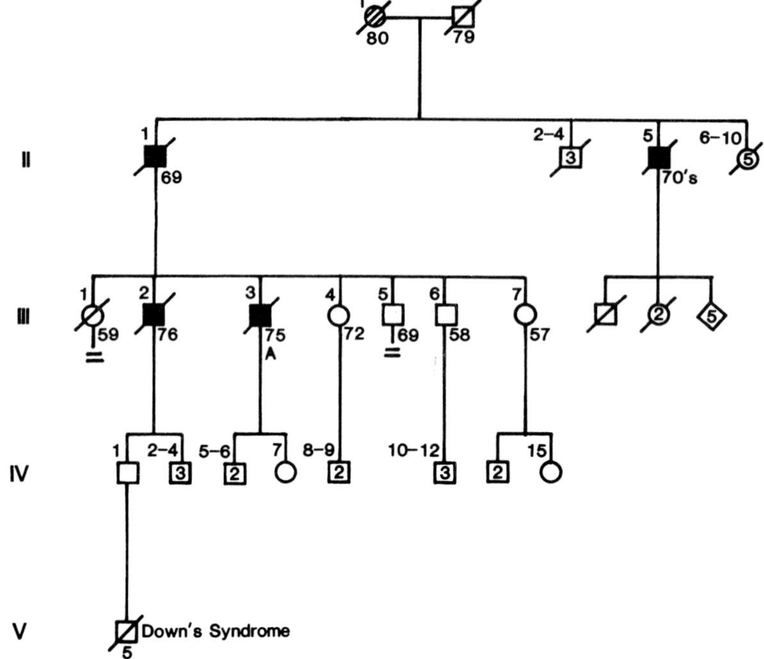

Fig. 6. The MMM family from the Belowesh colonies in the Ukraine. Autopsy (A) confirmed AD in III-3. For symbols, see Figure 2

man families because they all originated from the same two neighboring villages in Russia, they share several surnames and the disease is clinically and neuropathologically relatively uniform among the various kindreds. These families represent either a form of early-onset FAD or intermediate-onset FAD (Bird et al., 1990).

5. The Black Sea German families are likely to represent additional genetic heterogeneity. Compared to the Volga German kindreds, the Black Sea families come from different villages, generally have different surnames, tend to have smaller familial clusters of dementia and have a significantly later age of onset. The Black Sea German families seem to fit the classification of late-onset FAD.

Acknowledgments. Funded in part by NIH grant AG05136 and VA Medical Research Funds. Valuable help was provided by T. Kloberdanz, E. Reiswig, N. Zimmerer, J. Kissler, R. Haining, G. Glenner and E. Wilson.

References

Bird TD, Lampe TH, Nemens E, Miner G, Sumi S, Schellenberg G (1988) Familial Alzheimer's diseases in American descendants of the Volga Germans: Probable genetic founder effect. Ann Neurol 23:25–31

Bird TD, Sumi SM, Nemens EJ (1989) Phenotypic heterogeneity in familial Alzheimer's disease: A study of 24 kindreds. Ann Neurol 25:12–25

Bird TD, Hughes JP et al (1990) A proposed classification of familial Alzheimer's disease based on analysis of 32 multigeneration pedigrees. In: Maurer K, Riederer P, Beckmann H (eds) Key topics in brain research: Alzheimer's disease. Epidemiology, neurochemistry, and clinics. Springer-Verlag, Wien New York

Bird TD (1991) Evaluating family histories and traditions for evidence of medical illness using Alzheimer's disease as a model. Am Dis Soc Ger Russia J, pp 49–54

Cook RH, Ward BE, Austin JH (1979) Studies in aging of the brain: IV. Familial Alzheimer disease: Relation to transmissible dementia, aneuploidy, and microtubular defects. Neurology 29:1402–1412

Goate A, Chartier-Harlin MC, Mullan M, Brown J, Crawford F, Fidani L, Giuffra L, Haynes A, Irving N, James L, Mant R, Newton P, Rooke K, Roques P, Talbot C, Pericak-Vance M, Roses A, Williamson R, Rossor M, Owen M, Hardy J (1991) Segregation of a missense mutation in the amyloid precursor protein gene with familial Alzheimer's disease. Nature 349:704–706

Koch FC (1977) The Volga Germans in Russia and the Americas, from 1763 to the present. Pennsylvania State University Press, University Park and London

McKhann G, Drachman D, Folstein M, Katzman R, Price D, Stadlan EM (1984) Clinical diagnosis of Alzheimer's disease. Neurology 34:939–944

Mirra SS, Heyman A, McKeel D, Sumi SM, Crain BJ, Brownlee LM, Vogel FS, Hughes JP, van Behle G, Berg L (1991) The consortium to establish a registry for Alzheimer's disease (CERAD). Neurology 41:479–486

Risse SC, Lampe TH, Bird TD, Nochlin D, Sumi SM, Keenan T, Cubberley L, Peskind E, Raskind MA (1990) Myoclonus, seizures, and paratonia in Alzheimer's disease. Alz Dis Assoc Disorders 4:217–225

Sallet R (1974) Russian-German settlements in the United States. North Dakota Institute for Regional Studies, Fargo, ND

Schellenberg TD, Anderson L, O'Dahl S, Wijsman EM, Sadovnick AD, Ball MJ, Larson EB, Kukull WA, Martin GM, Roses AD, Bird TD (1991a) APP717, APP693, and PRIP gene mutations are rare in Alzheimer's disease. Am J Human Gen 49:511–517

Schellenberg GD, Pericak-Vance MA, Wijsman EM, Moore DK, Gaskell Jr PC, Yamaoka LA, Bebout JL, Anderson L, Welsh KA, Clark CM, Martin GM, Roses AD, Bird TD (1991b) Linkage analysis of familial Alzheimer's disease, using chromosome 21 markers. Am J Human Gen 49:563–583

Scheuerman RD, Trafzer CE (1985) The Volga Germans: Pioneers of the Northwest, University Press of Idaho, Moscow, ID

Protein Phosphorylation Regulates Processing of the Alzheimer β/A4-Amyloid Precursor Protein

S. E. Gandy, G. L. Caporaso, T. V. Ramabhadran,
J. D. Buxbaum, T. Suzuki, C. Nordstedt, K. Iverfeldt,
A. J. Czernik, A. C. Nairn, and P. Greengard

Introduction

Alzheimer's disease (AD) is the most common cause of primary brain failure, affecting approximately 10% of the over-65 population and 50% of the over-85 population. Clinically, early AD is characterized by prominent amnesia for recent events, while late AD is attended by a loss of much or all cerebral cortical function. Death typically occurs after six to eight years of illness, often due to a supvervening infection.

Neuropathologically, the brain affected by AD undergoes characteristic structural changes. Neuronal degeneration occurs in a typical pattern, prominently affecting the basal forebrain, the hippocampus and the association cortex (Price, 1986). Neurofibrillary tangles (NFT), apparently derived from normal cytoskeletal proteins that are abnormally phosphorylated (Sternberger et al., 1985; Grundke-Iqbal et al., 1986), develop within neurons. The role of the abnormal cytoskeletal phosphorylation in the pathogenesis of NFT is poorly understood, but evidence for a causal relationship has been presented (Hagstedt et al., 1989).

Outside brain cells, amyloid deposits form around gray matter blood vessels and within the cortical parenchyma. This particular amyloid peptide is unique to AD and related disorders, and is different from amyloid peptides associated with other systemic or organ-specific amyloidoses. All amyloids share the characteristic of "congophilia", referring to the ability of the precipitate to bind the dye Congo red. This property reflects a β-pleated sheet secondary structure, although the primary structures of the various amyloids are distinct.

In the mid-1980s, the Alzheimer amyloid deposits were discovered to be remarkably homogeneous in composition: greater than 90% of protein extractable from isolated vascular amyloid deposits (Glenner and Wong, 1984; "β protein") or from isolated parenchymal amyloid plaque cores (Masters et al., 1985; "A4 protein") yielded an identical sequence of about 40 amino acids. In 1987 and 1988, using oligonucleotide probes based upon the published sequence of the β/A4 protein, six laboratories (Kang et al., 1987; Goldgaber et al., 1987; Tanzi et al., 1987, 1988; Robakis et al., 1987; Ponte et al., 1988; Kitaguchi et al., 1988) reported the molecular cloning of several large transmembrane proteins (having isoforms of 695, 751, or 770 amino acids, generated

F. Boller et al. (Eds.)
Heterogeneity of Alzheimer's Disease
© Springer-Verlag Berlin Heidelberg 1992

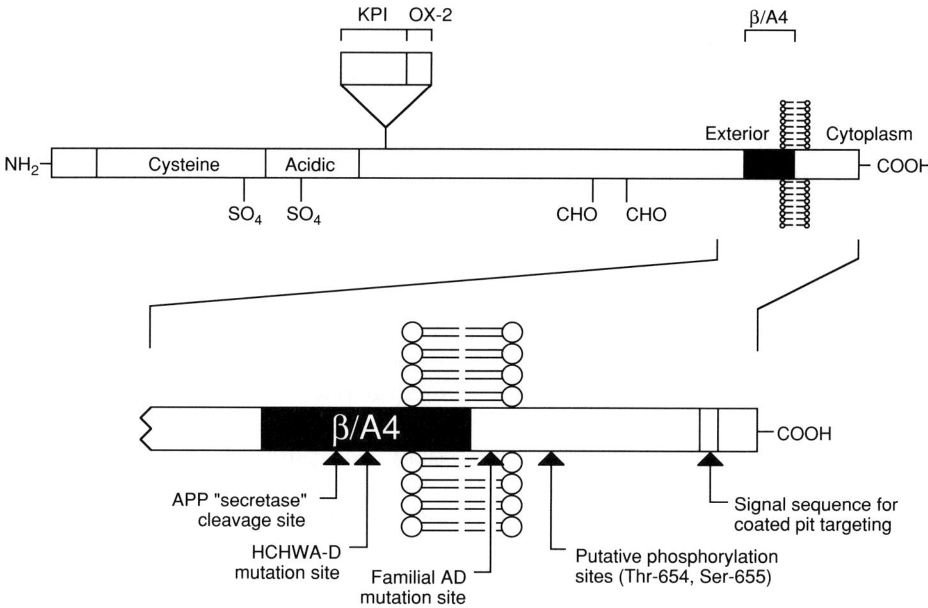

Fig. 1. Schematic diagram of the APP molecule

by alternative splicing of mRNA) that contained within them the sequence of the "β/A4 protein" and were thus named the Alzheimer, or β/A4, *a*myloid *p*recursor *p*roteins (APP; Fig. 1).

Phosphorylation of APP

Since abnormal protein phosphorylation had been implicated in the pathogenesis of NFT (Sternberger et al., 1985), the hypothesis was developed that aberrant protein phosphorylation might be a key event in the etiology of AD (Sternberger et al., 1985; Gandy et al., 1988). In our hypothesis, we suggested that a relationship might exist between abnormal protein phosphorylation and amyloidogenesis. The predicted cytoplasmic domain of APP contains amino acid sequences that resemble consensus sequences for serine, threonine or tyrosine protein phosphorylation. Therefore, we characterized the efficiency of short synthetic peptides containing these APP sequences to serve as substrates for phosphorylation, using either purified protein kinases or endogenous protein kinase activities from rat cerebral cortex (Gandy et al., 1988). Based on a comparison of kinetic parameters determined for the APP peptides with those for peptides corresponding to known physiological substrates, we identified an efficient site for phosphorylation of the APP cytoplasmic tail, located within a few amino acid residues from the plasma membrane. Protein kinase C (PKC) rapidly phosphorylates Ser^{655} (Kang et al., 1987; numbering for APP_{695}), whereas calcium/calmodulin-dependent protein kinase II rapidly phosphorylates Thr[654] and Ser[655] (Gandy et al., 1988). Recently, phosphorylation at the PKC site has been verified in studies using either a 50-amino acid synthetic peptide corresponding to the entire APP cytoplasmic domain (S. Gandy and P. Greengard, unpublished observations) or APP holoprotein (Suzuki et al., 1992). The APP holoprotein has also been demonstrated to be phosphorylated in cultures of intact human cells stably transfected with APP (Oltersdorf et al., 1990); the site of phosphorylation and the identity of the APP kinase responsible have not been determined.

The physiological effects of the phosphorylation of APP by protein kinase C may be anticipated based on the precedent studies of several transmembrane proteins. The epidermal growth factor receptor (EGFR; Beguinot et al., 1985; Lin et al., 1986) and the interleukin-2 receptor (IL-2R; Gallis et al., 1986; Shackelford et al., 1986) are integral phosphoproteins whose state of phosphorylation is regulated by PKC. The endocytosis of both EGFR and IL-2R is regulated by PKC-dependent phosphorylation. In addition, PKC is a potent regulator of the proteolytic processing of transforming growth factor-alpha (Pandiella and Massague, 1991) and the receptor for colony stimulating factor-1 (Downing et al., 1989). By analogy, we proposed that phosphorylation of APP by PKC might stimulate its internalization, and that this endocytic step might regulate the catabolism of APP and hence the process of amyloidogenesis. The endocytic pathway participates in processing of antigen molecules (Brodsky and Guagliardi, 1991) and might be particularly relevant to the APP processing which occurs at nerve terminals, since intact APP holoprotein undergoes rapid axonal transport (Koo et al., 1990) and is locally processed at the terminal (Sisodia et al., 1991).

Protein Phosphorylation and APP Processing

To test the effects of protein phosphorylation on APP metabolism, we prepared specific antibodies to study the biology of endogenous APP in PC-12 cells, an immortalized neuron-like cell line derived from a rat pheochromocytoma. These cells were chosen because of their neuronal lineage and because they express high levels of endogenous APP. Since the primary sequence of APP is highly conserved among many mammalian species, data obtained from studies of these cells may be relevant to our understanding of the biology of APP in human neurons.

Using [^{35}S]-methionine labeling in a pulse-chase protocol, we discovered that agents which regulate protein phosphorylation have dramatic effects on the proteolytic processing of APP (Buxbaum et al., 1990). Phorbol esters, which stimulate PKC, rapidly accelerate APP processing, generating a low molecular mass (15 kDa) carboxyl-terminal fragment of APP. Okadaic acid, a structurally unrelated compound that increases the state of protein phosphorylation by inhibiting two protein phosphatases (1 and 2A) that catalyze dephosphorylation reactions, appears to stimulate the generation of an identical fragment. When both agents are used together in a "hyperphosphorylation" paradigm, no further acceleration in production of the 15 kDa fragment is observed (as compared with either agent alone) but a slightly larger (19 kDa) fragment is recovered in addition to the 15 kDa species (Buxbaum et al., 1990).

Heterogeneity of APP Proteolysis

Coincident with our work on phosphorylation and APP processing, other groups (Sisodia et al., 1990; Esch et al., 1990) demonstrated that the normal proteolytic processing of APP (Weidemann et al., 1989; Oltersdorf et al., 1990) results in cleavage within the β/A4 domain, generating a 12 kDa carboxyl-terminal fragment, and thereby precludes amyloidogenesis. The current formulation is that the 15 kDa carboxyl-terminal fragment that we observe in PC-12 cells is identical to the 12 kDa fragment reported by others (Gandy et al., 1991a, 1992b; radiosequencing analysis, J. Buxbaum et al., unpublished observations). In addition, we speculate that the supraphysiological phosphorylation paradigm (phorbol plus okadaic acid) accelerates APP proteolysis to the point of saturating the "normal" intra-β/A4 cleavage pathway, and activates a minor pathway by default. This second pathway leads to cleavage at or near the NH_2-terminus of the β/A4 sequence, and thus represents a potentially amyloidogenic pathway of APP proteolysis (Gandy et al., 1991a, 1992a; Gandy and Greengard, 1992). High-level expression of human APP by recombinant vaccinia virus in CV-1 monkey fibroblast cells also yields electrophoretically heterogeneous APP carboxyl-terminal fragments in the 10–20 kDa range (Wolf et al., 1990). Presumably, in the vaccinia system, high-level expression provides supraphysiological levels of APP throughout the cell and leads to similar processing changes by virtue of inordinately high substrate concentration.

The basis for the electrophoretic microheterogeneity of APP carboxyl-terminal fragments is not yet fully understood, since heterogeneity of the site of cleavage (Buxbaum et al., 1990; Gandy et al., 1991a, 1992b), aggregation (Wolf et al., 1990), and/or alternative states of phosphorylation (see Steiner et al., 1990, for an example) may all be contributing factors. However, recent immunochemical characterizations of heterogeneous APP carboxyl-terminal fragments suggest that alternative (i.e., non-intra-β/A4 amyloid) cleavage of APP plays a role in generating the heterogeneity (Fig. 2). Specifically, potentially amyloidogenic carboxyl-terminal APP fragments (i.e., carboxyl-terminal APP fragments that are cleaved upstream of the standard intra-β/A4 site, and contain an intact β/A4-domain) have been identified in a number of laboratories. Moreover, evidence for the existence of these potentially amyloidogenic APP fragments has been obtained independently in several systems, including human cerebral vessels (Tamaoka and Selkoe, 1991; Levy and Frangione, 1991), human brain (Estus et al., 1992; Nordstedt et al., 1991), transfected human cells (Golde et al., 1991), and recombinant human APP-baculovirus infected Sf9 cells (Gandy et al., 1991b, 1992a). Purification and sequencing of potentially amyloidogenic APP carboxyl-terminal fragments is underway in all these laboratories. This line of research is perhaps the most promising lead in defining and characterizing the pathway to amyloid deposition.

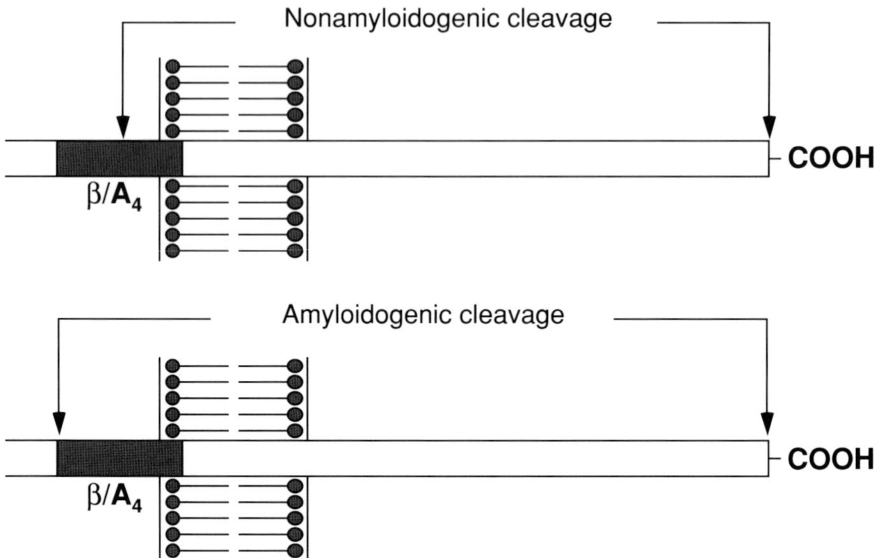

Fig. 2. Alternative proteolysis of APP: Nonamyloidogenic cleavage (upper) and potentially amyloidogenic cleavage (below)

In addition to the immunochemical evidence for alternative proteolysis of APP, radiosequence analyses of carboxyl-terminal fragments of APP generated in mammalian cells following vaccinia virus-mediated overexpression have provided preliminary evidence in support of alternative cleavage in that system (Higaki, Gandy, Greengard and Cordell, unpublished observations). Edman degradation analysis of a 15 kDa species labeled with [^{35}S]methionine yielded significant recovery of [^{35}S] radioactivity at cycle 19, consistent with standard (Esch et al., 1990) intra β/A4 processing, while other APP fragments of 16-, 17-, 22-, and 28-kDa, exhibited unique radiosequence profiles that are consistent with alternative sites of cleavage of APP. The apparent heterogeneity of APP processing observed in cultured mammalian cells following high-level expression with recombinant vaccinia virus (Wolf et al., 1990) led us to study APP processing following the infection of Spodoptera frugiperda (Sf9) cells with recombinant baculovirus bearing human APP. The baculoviral system facilitates the recovery and amino-terminal sequencing of APP fragment due to high levels of expression of recombinant proteins. APP$_{751}$ was selected for initial study because its overexpression was associated with the deposition of β/A4-amyloid in the brains of transgenic mice (Quon et al., 1991).

Immunochemical evidence for alternative cleavage of human APP$_{751}$ following high-level baculoviral overexpression has been reported (Gandy et al., 1991b, 1992a). The baculoviral overexpression of human APP$_{751}$ leads to the production of a limited number of discrete carboxyl-terminal fragments of 15 kDa, 16 kDa, 17 kDa and 25 kDa (Gandy et al., 1929a), apparently similar to the heterogeneous fragments identified in human tissues (Tamaoka and Selkoe, 1991; Estus et al., 1992; Nordstedt et al., 1991; Levy and Frangione, 1991) and

Table 1. Protein sequence of purified carboxyl-terminal APP_{751} fragments

Human APP/Sf9 cells	L V F F A X D V X X N X G A I I GL M V ...	(Ramabhadran et al., unpublished observations)
Human APP cDNA	...K L V F F A E D V G S N K G A I I GL M V ...	(Kang et al., 1987)
Human APP/human cells	X V F F A E D V G X ...	(Esch et al., 1990)

cultured human cells (Golde et al., 1991). Using the procedure of Esch et al. (1990), modified to include a final immunoaffinity chromatography step (employing affinity-purified and immobilized rabbit anti-human $APP^{645-694}$), the smallest human APP carboxyl-terminal species generated by Sf9 cells has been successfully purified and sequenced (Ramabhadran et al., manuscript in preparation). The sequence corresponds exactly to that which occurs in cleaved and secreted APP molecules following overexpression of human APP in human cells (Esch et al., 1990; Table 1).

These data provide evidence that the major APP cleavage is highly conserved throughout phylogeny. Furthermore, the recognition of this cleavage site by Sf9 cells enhances the usefulness and validity of the baculoviral system for the study of APP proteolysis. Complementary observations were recently reported by Lowery et al. (1991), who purified and sequenced the carboxyl-terminus of secreted APP ectodomain, also from the baculoviral system.

APP Mutations and Familial Cerebral Amyloidoses

Molecular genetics studies have strengthened the importance of APP processing in the pathogenesis of cerebral amyloidoses. Mutations in the coding sequence of APP associate with two distinct clinical and pathological phenotypes. Hereditary cerebral hemorrhage with amyloidosis of the Dutch-tyoe (HCHWAD) is an autosomal dominant disorder characterized by prominent cerebrovascular amyloidosis, relatively minor amyloidosis of brain parenchyma, and early mortality due to cerebral hemorrhage. HCHWAD apprears to be caused by a mutation within the β/A4 domain of APP (glutamate to glutamine at position 693 of APP_{770}), near the site of constitutive intra-amyloid cleavage (Levy et al., 1990; van Broeckhoven et al., 1990). This mutation presumably results in alteration of the post-translational modification and processing of APP, leading to defective, amyloidogenic processing and amyloid deposition (Selkoe, 1990).

The association of different mutant APP molecules with clinically typical familial Alzheimer's disease (FAD; Goate et al., 1991; Naruse et al., 1991; Murrell et al., 1991; Chartier-Harlin et al., 1991) suggests that abnormal disposition of APP or β/A4 may be both necessary and sufficient to cause full clinicopathological AD. These mutations, located within the APP transmembrane domain near its junction with the cytoplasmic domain, are rather conservative (valine to isoleucine, phenylalanine, or glycine, at position 717 of APP_{770}). The effects, therefore, are likely to be subtle, perhaps affecting conformation of the APP transmembrane or cytoplasmic domain and hence APP oligomerization with other integral proteins, APP proteolysis, APP phosphorylation, or APP interaction with intramembranous or cytosolic components (Gandy and Greengard, 1992b).

The identification of these mutations strongly suggests that the final common pathway in HCHWAD and FAD, and perhaps in the more typical sporadic type of AD, is disordered APP proteolysis and cerebral amyloidogenesis. This concept is consistent with reports of β/A4-amyloid neuroactivity (Whitson et al., 1989; Yankner et al., 1989, 1990; Flood et al., 1991; Kowall et al., 1991).

Cellular Routes for APP Processing

To completely understand the process of amyloidogenesis, substantially more information on cellular APP processing routes is required. Recently we have characterized two alternative trafficking and processing routes for some APP molecules.

In one study (Caporaso et al., 1992b), we obtained evidence that in PC-12 cells, only a minor population of molecules are targeted to the standard pathway for proteolytic cleavage within the β/A4-amyloid domain (Esch et al., 1990). Since this cleavage pathway is coupled to secretion of a large amino-terminal fragment, we have termed it the "standard secretory cleavage pathway". We have observed that the targeting of APP molecules to this standard pathway is regulated by protein phosphorylation, since either activation of PKC or inhibition of protein phosphatases 1 and 2A can independently accelerate the activity of the pathway. Figure 3 illustrates the effect of PKC activation on the generation of secreted amino-terminal fragments (Panel A) and on the generation of the cell-associated carboxyl-terminal fragment (Panel B).

In analyzing the products of the standard secretory cleavage pathway, we discovered that more than one-half of the molecules that were synthesized were apparently being degraded via a different route. Inhibitors of organelle function were used to dissect further the possible localization of APP degradation (Caporaso et al., 1992a). Brefeldin A, a compound that results in retention of newly synthesized molecules in the endoplasmic reticulum (ER), revealed no evidence for APP cleavage events occurring within the ER or early Golgi. Similar results were obtained with monensin, an ionophore whose effects include inhibition of distal Golgi function.

Additional studies along this line provided evidence for degradation of APP within an intracellular acidic vesicle (Caporaso et al., 1992a). Particularly useful was the weak base chloroquine, which acts to neutralize acidic intracellular organelles and thus to inhibit acid-dependent intravesicular proteolysis such as might occur in endosomes, lysosomes, and perhaps the trans-Golgi network.

Chloroquine had no effect on APP synthesis, maturation, or secretion (Fig. 4, panels A and B). This demonstrated that the drug did not exhibit generalized toxicity for the cells and that the standard secretory cleavage pathway was

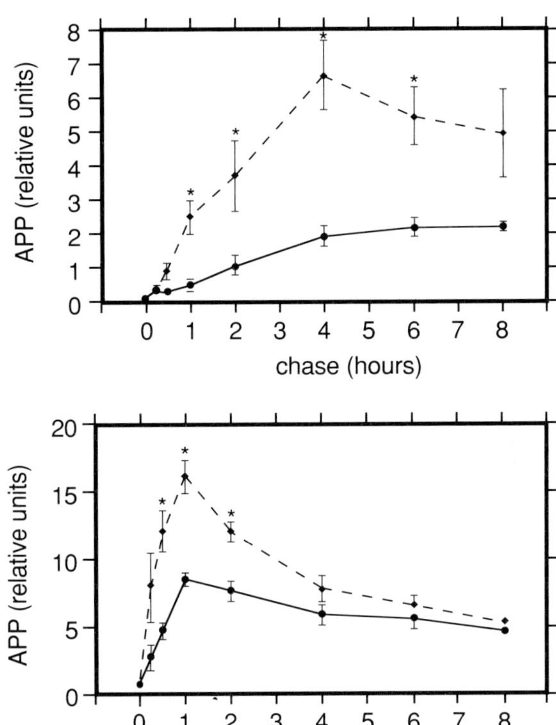

Fig. 3. Effects of PKC activation on the standard secretory cleavage of APP as determined by recovery of large secreted amino terminal fragment (panel A) and the low molecular weight cell-associated carboxyl-terminal fragment (panel B). Metabolism of APP species in the absence of phorbol ester (PDBu) is shown with solid lines and, in the presence of PDBu, with broken lines. Results shown in Panel A are for APP_{695}; similar results were obtained for APP_{751} and APP_{770} (from Caporaso et al., 1992b)

not substantially sensitive to intracellular intravesicular acidity. However, chloroquine dramatically diminished the intracellular degradation of mature APP holoprotein (Fig. 4, panel C). Furthermore, chloroquine inhibited the degradation of the small carboxyl-terminal fragment generated from cleavage of APP holoprotein in the standard secretory cleavage pathway (Fig. 4, panel D).

This series of experiments has allowed us to develop a scheme for the trafficking of APP molecules within the cell (Fig. 5). In this scheme, some mature APP molecules are targeted directly to a chloroquine-sensitive compartment for degradation, whereas others are targeted for intra-β/A4-amyloid cleavage and secretion in a pathway regulated by PKC and protein phosphatases 1 and 2A. Following secretory cleavage of mature APP, the carboxyl-terminal fragment thus generated is targeted to a chloroquine-sensitive compartment for degradation.

Definitive identification of which (if either) of these pathways can be a source for amyloidogenic carboxyl-terminal APP fragments has not yet been determined. This information is crucial to the successful dissection of the pathways of amyloidogenesis and to the design of strategies that will permit *in vitro* models of amyloidogenesis. It should be noted that cerebral amyloidosis is typically a late-life event, occurring after four or more decades of life. Thus,

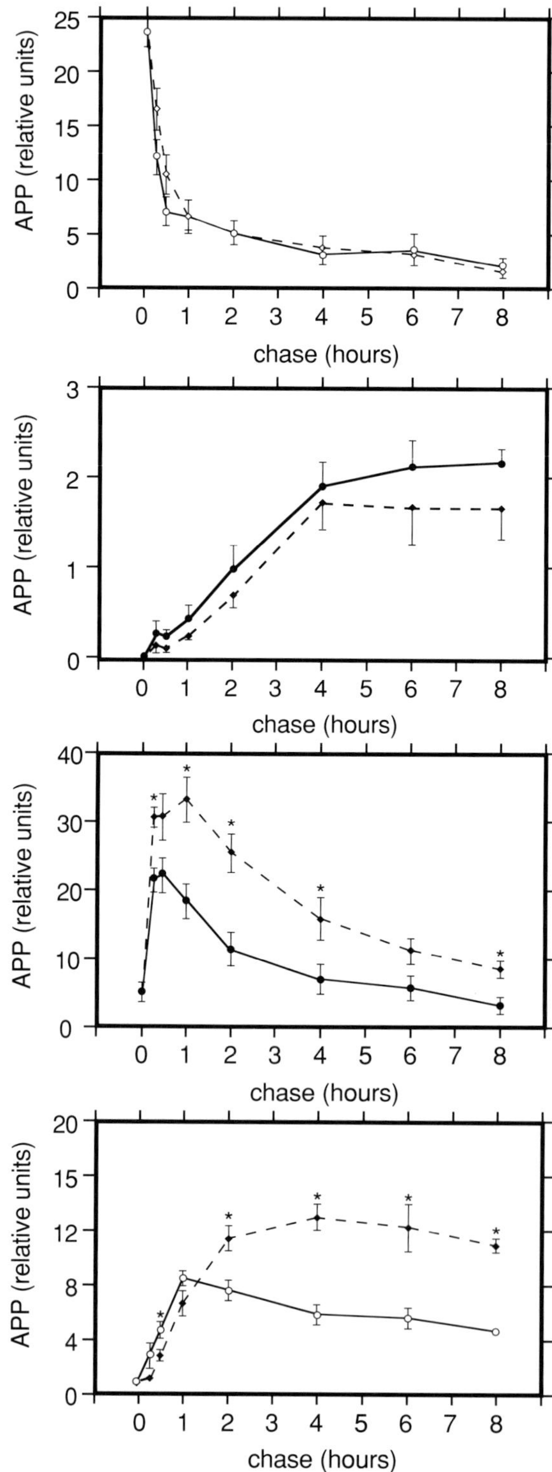

Fig. 4. Effects of chloroquine on the synthesis and maturation of APP (panel A), secretion of APP (panel B), intracellular degradation of mature APP (panel C) and intracellular degradation of the low molecular weight cell-associated carboxyl-terminal fragment of APP (panel D). Metabolism of APP species in the absence of chloroquine is shown with solid lines and in the presence of chloroquine with broken lines. Results shown in panels A, B, and C are for APP_{695}; similar results were obtained for APP_{751} and APP_{770} (from Caporaso et al., 1992a)

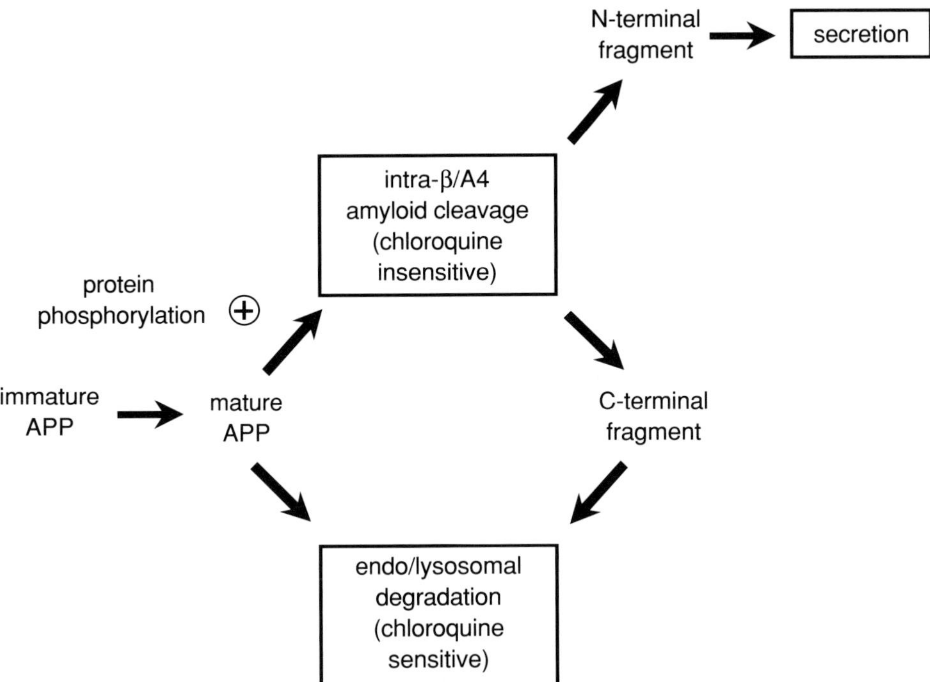

Fig. 5. Scheme for APP processing and its regulation

amyloidogenesis is likely to be an extremely low-grade process (Selkoe, 1991), even in the presence of amyloidogenic APP mutations which presumably enhance the fibrillogenic process.

Conclusions and Future Directions

The identification of alternative sites of cleavage is one step toward identification and isolation of the enzymes that catalyze amyloidogenic cleavage of APP, and the characterization of the regulation (perhaps by protein phosphorylation) of these enzymes. It seems likely that signal transduction via protein phosphorylation regulates the balance of the activities of these various pathways, some of which are nonamyloidogenic and others of which are likely to be amyloidogenic. In addition to defining the cleavage sites that generate amyloidogenic fragments, and identifying the proteases and protease inhibitors which regulate that cleavage, it will be of great interest to elucidate the signal transduction components that modulate the relative activities of the various pathways. It seems likely that disturbance of these signals may be relevant to the pathogenesis of AD, and particularly to the complex biochemical events that lead to the final common pathway of amyloidogenesis. Many of the components of these proteolytic and signal transduction systems (e.g., proteases cleaving APP, protein kinases and protein phosphatases acting on APP or APP proteases) may eventually serve as targets for rational drug therapy by antiamyloidogenic agents (Gandy and Greengard, 1992).

Acknowledgment. This work was supported by USPHS AG 09464 and AG 10491.

References

Beguinot L, Hanover JA, Ito S, Richert ND, Willingham MC, Pastan I (1985) Phorbol esters induce transient internalization without degradation of unoccupied epidermal growth factor receptors. Proc Natl Acad Sci USA 82:2774–2778

Brodsky FM, Guagliardi L (1991) The cell biology of antigen processing and presentation. Ann Rev Immunol 9:707–744

Buxbaum JD, Gandy SE, Cicchetti P, Ehrlich ME, Czernik AJ, Fracasso RP, Ramabhadran TV, Unterbeck AJ, Greengard P (1990) Processing of Alzheimer β/A4 amyloid precursor protein: Modulation by agents that regulate protein phosphorylation. Proc Natl Acad Sci USA 87:6003–6006

Caporaso GL, Gandy SE, Buxbaum JD, Greengard P (1992a) Chloroquine inhibits intracellular degradation but not secretion of Alzheimer β/A4 amyloid precursor protein. Proc Natl Acad Sci USA 89:2252–2256

Caporaso GL, Gandy SE, Buxbaum JD, Ramabhadran TV, Greengard P (1992b) Protein phosphorylation regulates secretion of Alzheimer β/A4 amyloid precursor protein. Proc Natl Acad Sci USA 89:3055–3059

Chartier-Harlin M, Crawford F, Houlden H, Warren A, Hughes D, Fidani L, Goate A, Rossor M, Roques P, Hardy J, Mullan M (1991) Early-onset Alzheimer's disease caused by mutations at codon 717 of the β-amyloid precursor protein gene. Nature 353:844–846

Downing JR, Roussel MF, Sherr CJ (1989) Ligand and protein kinase C downmodulate the colony stimulating factor 1 receptor by independent mechanisms. Mol Cell Biol 9:2890–2896

Esch FS, Keim PS, Beattie EC, Blacher RW, Culwell AR, Oltersdorf T, McClure D, Ward PJ (1990) Cleavage of amyloid β peptide during constitutive processing of its precursor. Science 248:1122–1124

Estus S, Golde T, Kunishita T, Blades D, Eisen M, Lowery D, Eisen M, Usiak M, Qu X, Tabira T, Greenberg B, Younkin S (1992) Potentially amyloidogenic, carboxyl-terminal derivatives of the amyloid protein precursor. Science 255:726–728

Flood J, Morley J, Roberts E (1991) Amnestic effects in mice of four synthetic peptides homologous to amyloid β-protein from patients with Alzheimer disease. Proc Natl Acad Sci USA 88:3363–3366

Gallis B, Lewis A, Wignall J, Alpert A, Mochizuki DY, Cosman D, Hopp T, Urdal D (1986) Phosphorylation of the human interleukin-2 receptor and a synthetic peptide identical to its C-terminal, cytoplasmic domain. J Biol Chem 261:5075–5080

Gandy S, Greengard P (1992) Amyloidogenesis in Alzheimer's disease: Some possible therapeutic opportunities. Trends Pharmacol Sci 13:108–113

Gandy SE, Czernik AJ, Greengard P (1988) Phosphorylation of Alzheimer disease amyloid precursor peptide by protein kinase C and calcium/calmodulin-dependent protein kinase II. Proc Natl Acad Sci USA 85:6218–6221

Gandy SE, Buxbaum JD, Greengard P (1991a) Signal transduction and the pathobiology of Alzheimer's disease. In: Iqbal K, Crapper-McLachlan D, Winblad B, Wisniewski HM (eds) Alzheimer's disease and related disorders. Wiley and Sons, New York, pp 155–172

Gandy SE, Bhasin R, Ramabhadran T, Koo E, Price D, Goldgaber D, Greengard P (1991b) Alzheimer β/A4 amyloid precursor protein: Evidence for putative amyloidogenic fragment. J Cell Biol 115:122a

Gandy SE, Bhasin R, Ramabhadran T, Koo E, Price D, Goldgaber D, Greengard P (1992a) Alzheimer β/A4 amyloid precursor protein: Evidence for putative amyloidogenic fragment. J Neurochem 58:383–386

Gandy SE, Buxbaum JD, Greengard P (1992b) A cell biological approach to the therapy of Alzheimer-type cerebral β/A4-amyloidosis. In: Khachaturian Z, Blass J (eds) Alzheimer's disease: new therapeutic strategies. Dekker, New York, pp 175–192

Glenner GG, Wong CW (1984) Alzheimer's disease: Initial report of the purification and characteristics of a novel cerebrovascular amyloid protein. Biochem Biophys Res Commun 122:885–890

Goate A, Chartier-Harlin M-C, Mullan M, Brown J, Crawford F, Fidani L, Guiffra L, Haynes A, Irving N, James L, Mant R, Newton P, Rooke K, Roques P, Talbot C, Pericak-Vance M, Roses A, Williamson R, Rossor M, Owen M, Hardy J (1991) Segregation of a missense mutation in the amyloid precursor protein gene with familial Alzheimer's disease. Nature 349:704–706

Golde T, Estus S, Younkin L, Usiak M, Younkin S (1991) C-terminal fragments containing full length β amyloid protein are produced during normal processing of the β amyloid protein precursor in cultured cells. Soc Neurosci Abstr 17:1293

Goldgaber D, Lerman MI, McBride OW, Saffioti U, Gajdusek DC (1987) Characterization and chromosomal localization of a cDNA encoding brain amyloid of Alzheimer's disease. Science 235:877–880

Grundke-Iqbal I, Iqbal K, Tung Y-C, Quinlan M, Wisniewski HM, Binder LI (1986) Abnormal phosphorylation of the microtubule-associated protein tau in Alzheimer cytoskeletal pathology. Proc Natl Acad Sci USA 83:4913–4917

Hagstedt T, Lichtenberg B, Wille H, Mandelkow E-M, Mandelkow E (1989) Tau protein becomes long and stiff upon phosphorylation: Correlation between paracrystalline structure and degree of phosphorylation. J Cell Biol 109:1643–1652

Kang J, LeMaire HG, Unterbeck A, Salbaum JM, Masters CL, Grzeschik KH, Multhaup G, Beyreuther K, Muller-Hill B (1987) The precursor of Alzheimer's disease amyloid A4 protein resembles a cell-surface receptor. Nature 325:733–736

Kitaguchi N, Takahashi Y, Tokushima Y, Shiojiri S, Ito H (1988) Novel precursor of Alzheimer's disease amyloid protein shows protease inhibitory activity. Nature 331:530–532

Koo EH, Sisodia SS, Archer DA, Martin LJ, Weidemann A, Beyreuther K, Masters CL, Fischer P, Price DL (1990) Precursor of amyloid protein in Alzheimer disease undergoes fast anterograde axonal transport. Proc Natl Acad Sci USA 87:1561–1565

Kowall N, Beal M, Busciglio J, Duffy L, Yankner B (1991) An in vivo model for the neurodegenerative effects of β-amyloid and protection by substance P. Proc Natl Acad Sci USA 88:7247–7251

Levy E, Carman MD, Fernandez-Madrid IJ, Power MD, Lieberburg I, van Duinen SG, Bots GTAM, Luyendik W, Frangione B (1990) Mutation of the Alzheimer's disease amyloid gene in hereditary cerebral hemorrhage, Dutch type. Science 248:1124–1126

Levy E, Frangione B (1991) Familial Alzheimer's disease. Current Biology 1:312–314

Lin CR, Chen WS, Lazar CS, Carpenter CD, Gill GN, Evans RM, Rosenfeld MG (1986) Protein kinase C phosphorylation at Thr 654 of the unoccupied EGF receptor and EGF binding regulate functional receptor loss by independent mechanisms. Cell 44:839–848

Lowery D, Pasternack J, Gonzalez-DeWitt P, Zurcher-Neely H, Tomich C, Altman R, Fairbanks M, Heinrikson R, Younkin S, Greenberg B (1991) Alzheimer's amyloid precursor protein produced by recombinant baculovirus expression: Proteolytic processing and protease inhibitory properties. J Biol Chem 266:19842–19850

Masters CL, Simms G, Weinmann NA, Multhaup G, McDonald BL, Beyreuther K (1985) Amyloid plaque protein in Alzheimer's disease and Down's syndrome. Proc Natl Acad Sci USA 82:4245–4249

Murrell J, Farlow M, Ghetti B, Benson M (1991) A mutation in the amyloid precursor protein associated with hereditary Alzheimer's disease. Science 254:97–99

Naruse S, Igarashi S, Kobayashi H, Aoki K, Inuzuka T, Kaneko K, Simizu T, Iihara K, Kojima T, Miyatake T, Tsuji S (1991) Mis-sense mutation Val-to-Ile in exon 17 of amyloid precursor protein gene in Japanese familial Alzheimer's disease. Lancet 337:978–979

Nordstedt C, Gandy S, Alafuzoff L, Caporaso G, Iverfeldt K, Grebb J, Winblad B, Greengard P (1991) Alzheimer β/A4-amyloid precursor protein in human brain: Aging-associated increases in holoprotein and in a proteolytic fragment. Proc Natl Acad Sci USA 88:8910–8914

Oltersdorf TL, Ward PJ, Henriksson T, Beattie EC, Neve RL, Lieberburg IL, Fritz LC (1990) The Alzheimer amyloid precursor protein: Identification of a stable intermediate in the biosynthetic/degradative pathway. J Biol Chem 265:4492–4497

Pandiella A, Massague J (1991) Cleavage of the membrane precursor for transforming growth factor alpha is a regulated process. Proc Natl Acad Sci USA 88:1726–1730

Ponte G, Gonzales-DeWhitt P, Schilling J, Miller J, Hsu D, Greenberg B, Davis K, Wallace W, Lieberburg I, Fuller F, Cordell B (1988) A new A4 amyloid mRNA contains a domain homologous to serine proteinase inhibitors. Nature 331:525–527

Price DL (1986) New perspectives on Alzheimer's disease. Ann Rev Neurosci 9:489–512

Quon D, Wang T, Catalano R, Scardina J, Cordell B (1991) Formation of β-amyloid protein deposits in brains of transgenic mice. Nature 352:239–241

Robakis NK, Ramakrishna N, Wolfe G, Wisniewski HM (1987) Molecular cloning and characterization of a cDNA encoding the cerebrovascular and the neuritic plaque amyloid peptides. Proc Natl Acad Sci USA 84:4190–4194

Selkoe DJ (1990) Deciphering Alzheimer's disease. The amyloid precursor protein yields new clues. Science 248:1058–1060

Selkoe DJ (1991) The molecular pathology of Alzheimer's disease. Neuron 6:487–498

Shackelford DA, Trowbridge IS (1986) Identification of lymphocyte integral membrane proteins as substrates for protein kinase. C J Biol Chem 261:8334–8341

Sisodia SS, Koo EH, Beyreuther K, Unterbeck A, Price DL (1990) Evidence that β-amyloid protein in Alzheimer's disease is not derived by normal processing. Science 248:492–495

Sisodia S, Koo E, Hoffman P, Koliatsos V, Perry G, Price D (1991) Fate of amyloid precursor protein in the nervous system. Soc Neurosci Abstr 17:1104

Steiner B, Mandelkow E-M, Biernat J, Gustke N, Meyer HE, Schmidt B, Mieskes G, Soling HD, Drechsel D, Kirschner MW, Goedert M, Mandelkow E (1990) Phosphorylation of microtube-associated protein tau: Identification of the site for calcium/calmodulin-dependent kinase and relationship with tau phosphorylation in Alzheimer tangles. EMBO J 9:3539–3544

Sternberger NH, Sternberger LA, Ulrich J (1985) Aberrant neurofilament phosphorylation in Alzheimer disease. Proc Natl Acad Sci USA 82:4274–4276

Suzuki T, Nairn A, Gandy S, Greengard P (1992) Phosphorylation of Alzheimer amyloid precursor protein by protein kinase C. Neuroscience, in press

Tamaoka A, Selkoe D (1991) Identification of a stable fragment of the Alzheimer amyloid precursor containing the intact β-protein in brain microvessels. Neurology 41 (Suppl 1):157

Tanzi R, Gusella JF, Watkins PC, Bruns GAP, St George-Hyslop P, Van Keuren ML, Patterson D, Pagan S, Kurnit DM, Neve RL (1987) Amyloid β protein gene: cDNA, mRNA distribution, and genetic linkage near the Alzheimer locus. Science 235:880–884

Tanzi R, McClatchey AI, Lamperti ED, Komaroff LV, Gusella JF, Neve RL (1988) Protease inhibitor domain encoded by an amyloid precursor mRNA associated with Alzheimer's disease. Nature 331:528–530

van Broeckhoven C, Haan J, Bakker E, Hardy JA, van Hul W, Wehnert A, Vegter-van der Vlis M, Roos RA (1990) Amyloid β-protein precursor gene and hereditary cerebral hemorrhage with amyloidosis, Dutch-type. Science 248:1120–1122

Weidemann A, Konig G, Bunke D, Fischer P, Salbaum JM, Masters CL, Beyreuther K (1989) Identification, biogenesis and localization of precursors of Alzheimer's disease A4 amyloid protein. Cell 57:115–126

Whitson JS, Selkoe DJ, Cotman CW (1989) Amyloid β-protein enhances the survival of hippocampal neurons in vitro. Science 243:1488–1490

Wolf D, Quon D, Wang Y, Cordell B (1990) Identification and characterization of C-terminal fragments of the β-amyloid precursor produced in cell culture. EMBO J 9:2079–2084

Yankner BA, Dawes LR, Fisher S, Villa-Komaroff L, Oster-Granite ML, Neve RL (1989) Neurotoxicity of a fragment of the amyloid precursor associated with Alzheimer's disease. Science 245:417–420

Yankner BA, Duffy LA, Kirschner DA (1990) Neurotrophic and neurotoxic effects of amyloid β-protein: Reversal by tachykinin neuropeptides. Science 250:279–282

Alzheimer's Disease and Neuroanatomy: Hypotheses and Proposals

C. Duyckaerts, P. Delaère, and *J.-J. Hauw*

Introduction

The advancement in the morphological understanding of Alzheimer's disease
has not paralleled the dramatic and recent improvement in our knowledge
concerning its biochemistry. Meanwhile, the value of morphological studies has
sometimes been underscored. In this paper, we would like to stress that Alzheimer's disease is not a general disorder that happens to affect the brain. Any
morphologist would agree that the lesions of Alzheimer's disease are "neural,"
involving neurons, synapses and pathways; some cortical areas are affected,
whereas other, immediately contiguous, areas are spared. The borders between
affected and spared areas are, most of the time, anatomical boundaries: Alzheimer's disease knows something about neuroanatomy. There are many ways
of explaining this propensity to comply with anatomical boundaries, and one of
the many possible ways of reading the neuropathological data has been
adopted here. It is not the only way to interpret the pathological data but it
may help to explain why a disease which may appear so heterogeneous from a
clinical point of view tends to be homogeneous pathologically: the extension of
the pathological process through specific anatomical pathways may indeed level
out lesions which might have been focal or regional at the onset of the disease.

Two abnormally processed proteins are involved in the pathogenesis of
Alzheimer's disease – β/A4 and tau – with two morphological counterparts –
neurofibrillary tangles and senile plaques. There are various ways of explaining
these morphological changes (Fig. 1). One may consider that they are bystanders to a biochemical process, the course of which determines the course of
the disease (biochemical point of view). By contrast, one may believe that
these lesions are directly involved in the pathological process (morphological
point of view). Neuropathologists are inclined to adopt this latter point of view,
which has been presented in various studies and reviews (Pearson et al., 1985;
Rogers and Morrison, 1985; Duyckaerts et al., 1986; Mann, 1988; Hauw et al.,
1990) and which we shall also follow.

If plaques and tangles are directly implicated in the pathogenesis of the
disease, then we should try to explain how the process progresses from a
relatively circumscribed disease, confined to the hippocampus, to a widespread
disorder involving associative cortices and subcortical nuclei. There are probably no other neurological diseases which exhibit such an orderly progression:

F. Boller et al. (Eds.)
Heterogeneity of Alzheimer's Disease
© Springer-Verlag Berlin Heidelberg 1992

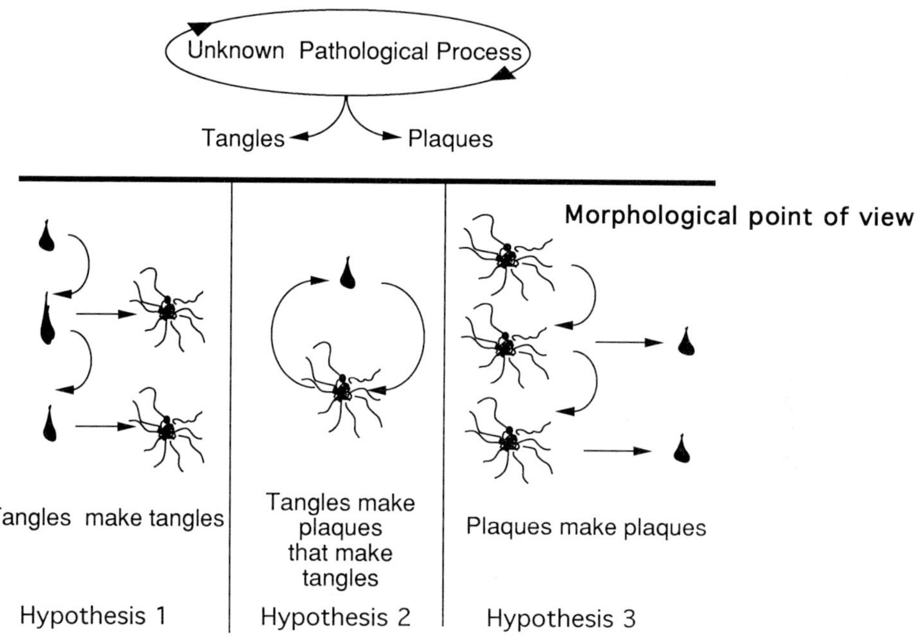

Fig. 1. Ways of viewing Alzheimer's pathology. Diagram intended to schematically character-ize the various ways of viewing the significance of Alzheimer's pathology. From the "bio-chemical point of view," the morphological lesions are just bystanders or markers of a pathological process which, itself, remains invisible. From the "morphological point of view," the lesions are, themselves, the agents of the disease process. Three possibilites may explain the progression of the disease: the presence of tangles induces the formation of new tangles (hypothesis 1); the presence of plaques induces the formation of new plaques (hypothesis 3); or, finally, one lesion may induce the formation of the other (hypothesis 2). We favor this latter hypothesis (see text for explanation)

Pick's disease is, often for a long time, limited to one lobe. The brunt of Huntington's chorea is on the striatum and the cortical alterations remain relatively light, even in severe cases. In Parkinson's disease, only a few cases exhibit a large number of Lewy bodies in the cortex. We believe that the progressive involvement of the cortex occurring in Alzheimer's disease is pecu-liar to this disorder and is a clue to its understanding. Moreover, this progres-sion of the disease process contrasts with the limited involvement of the brain in so-called normal aging (Hauw et al., 1988).

Adopting the "morphological point of view" mentioned earlier, we can imagine several ways by which lesions multiply. Tangles may be at the origin of new tangles; in this case, plaques would not play any role in the diffusion of the disease to other parts of the cortex (hypothesis 1 of Fig. 1). Following the opposite view, plaques could generate new plaques; the tangles, this time, would be the bystanders (hypothesis 3 of Fig. 1). Finally, one could imagine an interaction between plaques and tangles: plaques could generate tangles, which would induce an upsurge of new plaques (or, in a similar manner, tangles would make plaques, which would make tangles; there is no hint as to what comes first, plaques or tangles). This last hypothesis (hypothesis 2 of Fig. 1) is, in our view, more parsimonious and in better accordance with several facts. We do not know of cases which are devoid of plaques or of tangles; both these lesions are present. Although plaques may sometimes be the only lesions in the neocortex (Terry et al., 1987), tangles are always found in the hippocampus.

β/A4 deposits, tangle-bearing neurons and clinical signs

Before elaborating on these hypotheses of how the disease process expands throughout the brain, we would like first to consider three hard facts which should be included in any type of hypothesis that tries to explain how the disorder progresses within the brain.

1. So-called pre-amyloid (Tagliavini et al., 1988; Bugiani et al., 1989), diffuse β/A4 deposits are not responsible for the clinical signs. We have, indeed, observed one case of a prospectively assessed, intellectually normal individual who had massive deposition of β/A4 protein in the brain (Delaère et al., 1990). In that case, the deposits were not impairing the intellectual functions. Similar observations lead Dickson et al. (1991) to isolate a group of "pathological aging" among intellectually normal individuals. These data are in accordance with the observations that the distribution of βA4 deposits in the brain is rather unspecific and diffuse (Arnold et al. 1991).

2. The clinical signs are better explained by tangle pathology, i.e., neurofibrillary tangles in the perikaryon, neuropile threads (Braak et al., 1986; Duyckaerts et al., 1989), and neuritic component of the senile plaque. In our clinicopathological studies, the correlation between the Blessed test score and the pathology is always high when neurofibrillary stains, such as Bodian's method or tau immunostain, are used (Duyckaerts et al., 1987; Delaère et al., 1989; Lamy et al., 1989).

3. Not all the neurons are prone to exhibit tangles. Some are spared, including the small neurons, such as the granule cells of layer IV, or the very large neurons, such as the Betz cells in the motor cortex or the Purkinje cells in the cerebellum. The most often involved neurons are the medium-sized pyramidal neurons in the hippocampus and neocortex and the medium-sized multipolar neurons in the subcortical nuclei.

Alzheimer's disease knows something about neuroanatomy

The progression of Alzheimer's disease follows anatomical pathways; there are several examples of the compliance of the disease to neuroanatomy. We would like to expand upon two of them: the distribution of neuritic plaques and the topography of the changes in the hippocampus.

Distribution of neuritic plaques

We (Duyckaerts et al., 1986) as well as others (Rogers et al., 1985; Pearson et al., 1985) noticed that neuritic plaques (i.e., plaques made of an amyloid center and a crown of degenerating neurites) are not distributed at random. In the cerebral neocortex, they are mainly located in a band which lies midway between the pial surface and the white matter, corresponding to layer III. This region is supposed to be involved in cortico-cortical connections (Gilbert, 1985). Tangential sections of flat-mounted cortex reveal a non-random, regular distribution of the plaques, suggesting the degeneration of regularly spaced projecting fibers (unpublished data).

Distribution of the lesions in the hippocampus

According to a well-accepted view (Pandya and Seltzer, 1982; Mesulam, 1985), the hippocampus is at the focus of converging afferent connections coming from multimodal associative cortices. Fibers coming from those cortices connect with the neurons of the entorhinal cortex. From the entorhinal cortex, the perforant path crosses the subiculum and synapses with the neurons of the dentate gyrus, which in turn give off the mossy fibers. Those are connected with the CA3 pyramidal neurons (see, for example, Amaral, 1987).

Numerous tangles are visible in the entorhinal cortex (Fig. 2), even in the less severely affected cases (Hyman et al., 1984; Braak and Braak, 1985, 1991). The perforant path partially degenerates (Hyman et al., 1986). A row of senile plaques is laid along the dentate gyrus and these probably include fibers of the perforant path. The neurons of the dentate gyrus, being granule cells, do not develop tangles (see above) and the mossy fibers (axons of the dentate granule cells) are spared. There are almost no tangles or plaques in the CA3 sector. We believe that they are absent because the sequence of pathological events is interrupted by the presence of the resistant granule cells, which stop the process of plaque and tangle formation within a chain of synaptically connected regions. This contrasts with the CA1 sector, which is massively connected with the entorhinal area and is severely involved by Alzheimer's pathology (see, for review, Saper, 1988). The compliance of the disease to neuroanatomy is, in our view, due to the fact that the lesions are not independent from the neurons themselves; they are in fact connected with the nervous network.

How are the senile plaques connected with the nervous tissue?

There is evidence that the plaques are not "extra-neural" lesions such as inflammatory cells or amorphous deposits; silver impregnation shows the presence of neurites and electron microscopy (Terry et al., 1964; Foncin and Lebeau, 1965), shows presynaptic endings in the crown of the plaques. Immunostain reveals tau epitopes (Brion et al., 1985; Delaère et al., 1989). Synaptophysin antigen, a marker of pre-synaptic endings, is present even in diffuse

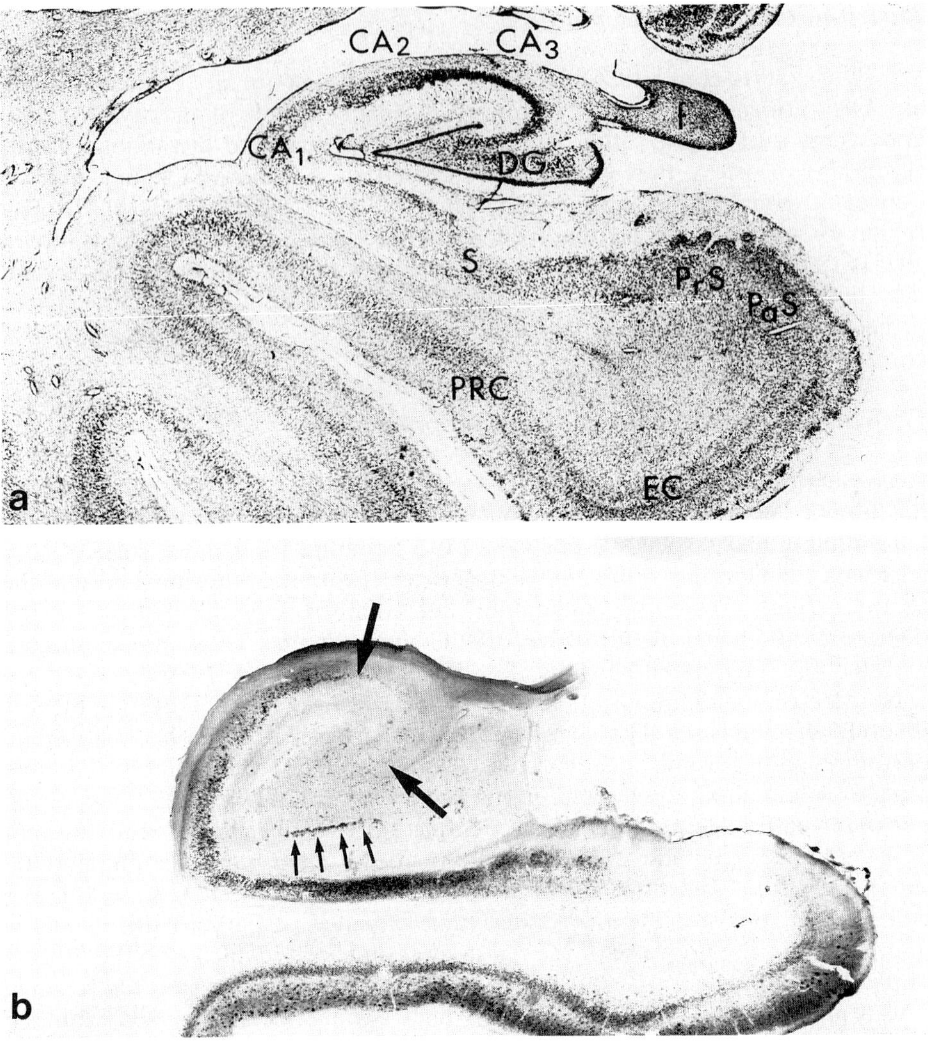

Fig. 2a, b. Hippocampal pathology. *a*; Map of the human hippocampal regions from Amaral (1987, with permission), Nissl stain. DG, dentate gyrus; S, subiculum; PrS, presubiculum; PaS, parasubiculum; EC, entorhinal cortex; PRC, perirhinal cortex. *b*, Alzheimer's lesions stained by Gallyas technique on 100 μm thick vibratome section. The neurofibrillary tangles and the plaque crowns are stained in black. Small arrows, row of plaques in the molecular layer of the dentate gyrus. Big arrows, relative sparing of the CA3 sector, which appears white in comparison to the rest of the cortex

deposits (Bugiani et al., 1990; Brion et al., 1991). These techniques, however, do not uncover the relationship of the plaques with the neurons and indeed, we do not know which neurons are connected to the senile plaques. Golgi methods which impregnate a few neurons in their entirety have been used to describe the interface between the plaques and the nervous system (Probst et al., 1983).

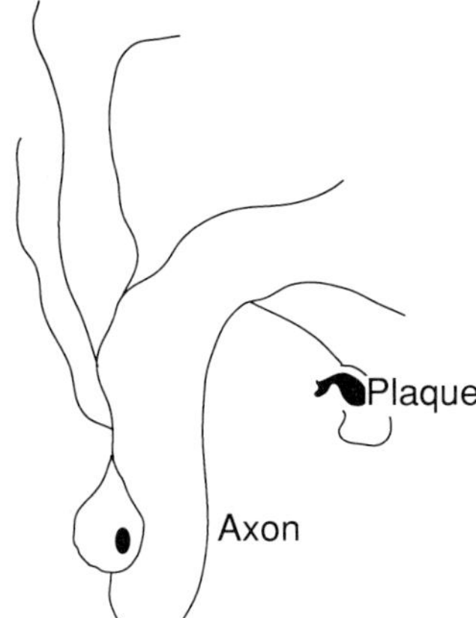

Fig. 3. Hypothetical way that a plaque attracts an axon. Several lines of evidence suggest that the senile plaques ("plaque") are innervated by presynaptic endings ("axons"). The radiating aspect of the nervous processes in contact with the plaque core is highly suggestive of an attraction of the nervous processes by the plaques, as shown in this drawing

However, with the usual Golgi techniques, plaques are covered by a clump of precipitates which are difficult to distinguish from artefacts. To better apprehend the structure of plaques with Golgi technique, we partially disimpregnated the section and restained it with various methods. Our results were unsatisfactory with immunostain and thioflavin S, but some silver techniques gave interesting (although preliminary), results. By counterstaining the deimpregnated section with Bodian's method, we could recognize and examine Golgi-impregnated senile plaques. Most of the neurites which were converging toward the center of the plaques were indeed axons. We found that some dendrites could participate in the plaque innervation, but they were rare; most of the time, the course of the dendrite, even if it crossed a plaque, was not affected. The sprouting of dendrites, around the plaque, was rarely seen but, on the other hand, numerous axons, often of small diameter and sometimes of beaded appearance, were coursing to the plaque, sometimes altering their course to reach it. We believe that the only way of explaining the radiating appearance of the plaques is to admit that the plaque itself attracts axons (Fig. 3). Several explanations of this hypothetical attraction come to mind: β/A4 protein could act by chemotactism or the formation of an amyloid precipitate could immobilize other chemotactic substances. We have to remember, however, that several amyloid deposits (particularly in prion's disease) do not attract neurites. This finding probably suggests that β/A4 protein itself plays a major role in the process (Duyckaerts et al., 1988). On the other hand, numerous β/A4 deposits are not surrounded by degenerating neurites; most of the cerebellar and striatal deposits, for example, are devoid of neurites. This suggests that the deposits do not attract all axons, but only a subset of them. It is also probable that the plaque cannot attract an axon at a great distance from its synaptic ending; it is more plausible that only the axonal endings which are located nearby are attracted by the plaques. Golgi impregnation rarely shows (Probst et al., 1983), and never in our material, the innervation of the plaques by nearby neurons; only exceptional axons, coming from the plaque, can be

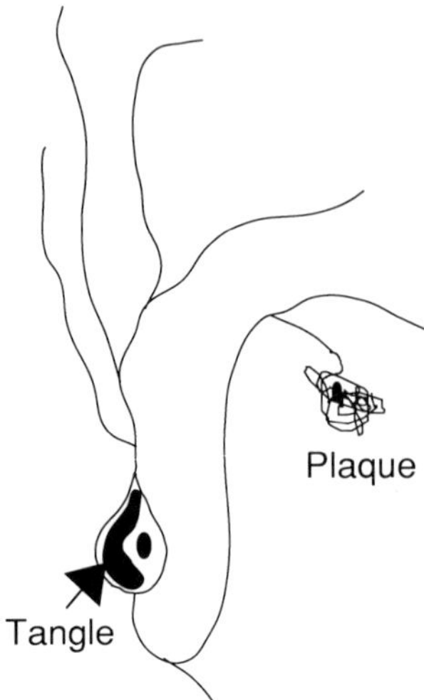

Fig. 4. Hypothetical mechanism for the spreading of Alzheimer's pathology: a neuron in contact with a plaque develops a tangle. It is not known if neurons in synaptic contacts with plaques are themselves altered and exhibit tangles. We have pursued this possibility, which is part of hypothesis 2 ("plaques make tangles," see Fig. 1) and which is sketched here. A neuron in contact with a plaque has secondarily developed a tangle

traced to a neuron (in the limits of 100 μm thick, Golgi-impregnated section). This leads us to conclude that plaques are mostly innervated by neurons which are located relatively far away from them.

These data demonstrate that the plaques are connected to the nervous tissue by axons. It is then tempting to imagine that (some? all?) neurons connected to the plaque by their axons are, in turn, altered. Let us accept, for the sake of our hypothesis, that those neurons which have axonal connections with plaques develop tangles in their perikarya (Fig. 4). Some evidence supports this assumption; as already noticed by German et al. (1987), it is noteworthy that many subcortical nuclei whose neurons are prone to develop tangles are those which are directly connected with the cerebral cortex. This may be compatible with the retrograde degeneration of the neurons in contact with the plaques pathology present in the neocortex. This point leads us to the next question.

How are the tangle-bearing neurons connected?

Extra-cellular tangles ("ghost tangles") are often observed, especially in the hippocampus. This has lead to the belief that the tangle kills the neurons in which it develops (Saper et al., 1985). Confirming this possibility is the good concordance between the type of neurons that disappear during the disease (Terry et al., 1981) and those that bear tangles in their perikaryon. Although there are exceptions to this concordance (e.g., the retina; Hinton et al., 1986), most neuropathologists would probably agree that tangles produce cell loss. We believe, however, that it would be a mistake to consider that tangle-bearing neurons are "tombstones" marking a process which has taken place long before; what happens to the processes of a neuron whose perikaryon is filled with a tangle is not well understood. The Golgi method is the most readily available technique to clarify this point, but unfortunately, tangles are incon-

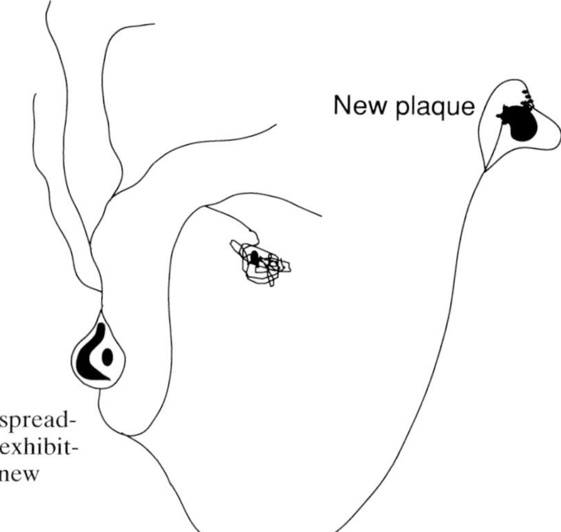

Fig. 5. Hypothetical mechanism for the spreading of Alzheimer's pathology: a neuron exhibiting a tangle initiates the formation of a new plaque

spicuous in Golgi-impregnated material. To detect those tangle-bearing neurons, we de-impregnated the Golgi-Cox stained section and re-stained it with Gallyas method. We recognized tangles in a few neurons. Their dendritic tree was still clearly visible, well-developed and devoid of any significant morphological alterations. Gertz et al. (1991) mentioned that the dendritic harbor of a tangle-bearing neuron may be quite large. Unfortunately, we have no information concerning the axonal process of those neurons but, since the presence of a tangle is compatible, at least for a certain time, with the survival of a "full-blown" neuron, we conclude that its axon can keep its normal course, at least for a certain amount of time. This would imply that the axon of a tangle-bearing neuron might reach some regions located far from the affected perikaryon. Endorsing hypothesis 2 ("plaques make tangles that make plaques"), we then imagine that the degeneration of the terminal part of this axon is at the origin of a new plaque (Fig. 5). There is no clear evidence for this assumption, but it seems reasonable to believe that plaques and tangles somehow interact in the spreading of the disease; otherwise there should be cases with only one type of lesions, to the exclusion of the other.

A network of lesions

If plaques and tangle-bearing neurons are connected, then the lesions involve a network that covers the cortex; the next question would be, "where does it start within that network?" Braak and Braak (1991) developed a staging of the lesions based on the alterations observed in the entorhinal and hippocampal cortices. This staging assumes that the lesions spread over the cortex in a stepwise manner. Cases from our prospectively assessed cohort (Charles Foix longitudinal study) were staged by Braak (unpublished observations) and the result of this staging was compared to the density of the neocortical β/A4 deposits (Delaère et al., 1991). We found that the hippocampal stage could already demonstrate a marked involvement in cases where the neocortex was still devoid of any βA4 deposits. This suggests that the hippocampal pathology precedes the neocortical lesions and strengthens the assumption that Alzheimer's disease starts in the limbic system. On the other hand, the entorhinal prominence of the lesions could be due to the convergence of the cortico-cortical pathways on the limbic systems. By following the anatomical paths, as here hypothesized, lesions would be concentrated in the limbic system. If this were the case, then a very large area of the neocortex would have to be screened to obtain the same amount of lesions as seen in a restricted area of the hippocampus. This "lesion concentration" effect would readily explain why the limbic pathology of Alzheimer's disease is so similar from case to case, even though clinical signs might be different at the beginning of the disease (aphasia, apraxia, hemiplegia; making up the group of so-called "focal Alzheimer's disease"). Wherever the disorder starts, it spreads along the same network, which it fills with lesions; at the end, the pathological picture is strikingly homogeneous. This hypothesis would predict that the sampling of very large areas of the neocortex would show a few definite lesions at stages where the hippocampus would already be markedly affected.

Functioning of altered cortices

Patients with extensive Alzheimer's pathology retain the ability to walk around; they are not blind, deaf or mute, although their cognitive functions are deeply altered. This indicates that the neocortex, even with severe Alzheimer's changes, retains some of its functioning capabilites. The dissection, performed by the pathological process, of the cortical abilities in immediate action and sensation (walking, hearing, etc.) from the cognitive processes (going somewhere, understanding, etc.) is surprising and can not be understood purely in terms of affected versus spared areas. It is indeed clear, even at the early stages of the disease, that very large areas of the cortex, including sensorimotor and primary associative cortices, are implicated. We tend to believe that, within each area of the cortex, some systems are more involved in immediate sensations and actions and are resistant to the Alzheimer's pathological process (Fig. 6). Other systems (involving middle-sized pyramidal neurons) are more dedicated to cognitive and memory functions and converge onto the perirhinal, entorhinal and hippocampal cortices; these "memory neurons" may be more sensitive to Alzheimer's pathology, exhibit tangles and produce plaques.

Conclusions

We have developed hypotheses concerning the development of Alzheimer's lesions along neuroanatomical pathways. Our main aim was to pinpoint a fact which should not be underestimated: the distribution of plaques and tangles follows neuroanatomy in many aspects. Plaques are innervated by axons whose origins remain unclear. Tangles affect some specific types of neurons; the projection of these neurons and the effect of their lesions on the cells with which they are connected remain unknown.

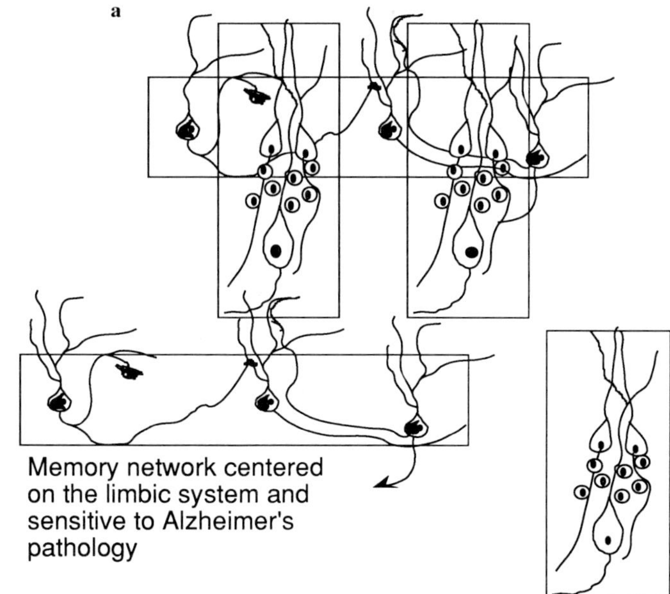

Fig. 6a–c. Dissection of brain functions by Alzheimer's pathology. A brain severely affected by Alzheimer's pathology retains some of its functions (even severely affected patients can walk around; they are not blind, deaf or mute). This cannot be fully understood in terms of regional topography. Even affected cortical areas seem to retain some of their functions. This fact is used as a basis for the following hypothetical dichotomy. The cortex (*a*) would include two distinct sets of neurons, some of which would be assigned to memory functions (*b*), centered on the limbic system (memory neurons), and some of which would be involved in immediate (motor or sensory) actions (actuators and sensors; *c*). The first type of neuron would be sensitive to Alzheimer's pathology, whereas the second type would be resistant

The isolation of a mutation of the amyloid precursor protein (APP) gene in some families strongly suggests that the APP by itself may trigger the disease. This important finding, however, stresses our ignorance of the mechanisms which link the gene and the disease (Hardy and Higgins, 1992). How can it be that such a diffusely distributed abnormality of APP metabolism leads to a disease which affects only specific neurons, layers, nuclei, etc., in a very stereotyped way? New hypotheses and new methods to test them (among which are techniques to track connections) should help to determine why, indeed, "Alzheimer's disease knows something about neuroanatomy".

References

Amaral DG (1987) Memory: anatomical organization of candidate brain regions. In: Mountcastle VB, Plum F, Geiger SR (eds) Handbook of physiology. The nervous system. Section 1. Williams & Wilkins, Baltimore, pp 211–294

Arnold SE, Hyman BT, Flory J, Damasio AR, van Hoesen GW (1991) The topographical and neuroanatomical distribution of neurofibrillary tangles and neuritic plaques in the cerebral cortex of patients with Alzheimer's disease. Cerebral Cortex 1:103–116

Braak H, Braak E (1985) On areas of transition between temporal allocortex and temporal isocortex in the human brain. Normal morphology and lamina specific pathology in Alzheimer's disease. Acta Neuropathol 68:325–332

Braak H, Braak E (1991) Neuropathological stageing of Alzheimer-related changes. Acta Neuropathol (Berl) 80:479–486

Braak H, Braak E, Grundke-Iqbal I, Iqbal K (1986) Occurrence of neuropil threads in the senile human brain and in Alzheimer's disease: a third location of paired helical filaments outside neurofibrillary tangles and senile plaques. Neurosci Lett 65:351–355

Brion J-P, Passareiro H, Nunez J, Flament-Durand J (1985) Mise en évidence immunologique de la protéine tau au niveau des lésions de dégénérescence neurofibrillaire de la maladie d'Alzheimer. Arch Biol 95:229–235

Brion J-P, Couck A-M, Bruce M, Anderton B, Flament-Durand J (1991) Synaptophysin and chromogranin A immunoreactivities in senile plaques of Alzheimer's disease. Brain Res 539:143–150

Bugiani O, Giaccone G, Frangione B, Ghetti B, Tagliavini F (1989) Alzheimer's patients: preamyloid deposits are more widely distributed than senile plaques throughout the central nervous system. Neurosci Lett 103:263–268

Bugiani O, Giaccone G, Verga L, Pollo B, Ghetti B, Frangione B, Tagliavini F (1990) Alzheimer patients and Down patients: abnormal presynaptic terminals are related to cerebral preamyloid deposits. Neurosci Lett 119:56–59

Delaère P, Duyckaerts C, Brion J-P, Poulain V, Hauw J-J (1989) Tau, PHF, and amyloid in the neocortex, a morphometric study of 15 cases with graded intellectual status in aging and SDAT. Acta Neuropathol (Berlin) 77:645–653

Delaère P, Duyckaerts C, Masters C, Piette F, Hauw J-J (1990) Large amounts of neocortical A4 deposits without Alzheimer lesions in a psychometrically-assessed non demented person. Neurosci Lett 116:87–93

Delaère P, Duyckaerts C, He Y, Piette F, Hauw J-J (1991) Subtypes and differential laminar distribution and of βA4 deposits in Alzheimer's disease: relationship with intellectual status in 26 cases. Acta Neuropathol (Berlin) 81:328–335

Dickson D, Crystal HA, Mattiace LA, Masur DM, Blau AD, Davies P, Yen SH, Aronson MK (1991) Identification of normal and pathological aging in prospectively studied non-demented elderly humans. Neurobiol Aging 13:179–189

Duyckaerts C, Hauw J-J, Bastenaire F, Piette F, Poulain C, Rainsard V, Javoy-Agid F, Berthaux P (1986) Laminar distribution of neocortical senile plaques in senile dementia of the Alzheimer type. Acta Neuropathol (Berlin) 70:249–256

Duyckaerts C, Brion J-P, Hauw J-J, Flament-Durand J (1987) Quantitative assessment of the density of neurofibrillary tangles and senile plaques in senile dementia of the Alzheimer type. Comparison of immunocytochemistry with a specific antibody and Bodian's protargol method. Acta Neuropathol (Berlin) 73:167–170

Duyckaerts C, Delaère P, Poulain V, Brion J-P, Hauw J-J (1988) Does amyloid precede paired helical filaments in the senile plaque? A study of 15 cases with graded intellectual status in aging and Alzheimer disease. Neurosci Letters 91:354–359

Duyckaerts C, Kawasaki H, Delaère P, Rainsard C, Hauw J-J (1989) Fiber disorganisation due to kinked fibers in the neocortex of patients with senile dementia of the Alzheimer type. Neuropath Appl Neurobiol 15:233–247

Foncin JF, Lebeau J (1965) Ultrastructure des plaques séniles. Rev Neurol (Paris) 112:61–62

German DC, White CL, Sparkman DR (1987) Alzheimer's disease: neurofibrillary tangles in nuclei that project to the cerebral cortex. Neuroscience 21:305–312

Gertz HJ, Krüger H, Patt S, Cervos-Navarro J (1991) Tangle-bearing neurons show more extensive dendritic trees than tangle-free neurons in area CA1 of the hippocampus in Alzheimer's disease. Brain Res 548:260–266

Gilbert CD (1985) Horizontal integration in the neocortex. Trends Neurosci 8:160–165

Hardy JA, Higgins GA (1992) Alzheimer's disease: the amyloid cascade hypothesis. Science 256:184–185

Hauw J-J, Duyckaerts C, Delaère P (1988) Neuropathology of aging and SDAT: how can age-related changes be distinguished from those due to disease process? In: Henderson AS, Henderson JH (eds) Etiology of dementia of Alzheimer type. Dahlem Konferenzen, London, pp 195–211

Hauw J-J, Duyckaerts C, Delaère P, Piette F (1990) Topography of lesions in Alzheimer's disease: a challenge to morphologists. In: Rapoport SI, Petit H, Leys D, Christen Y (eds) Imaging, cerebral topography and Alzheimer's disease. Springer Verlag, Berlin, pp 53–67

Hinton DR, Sadun AA, Blanks JC, Miller CA (1986) Optic-nerve degeneration in Alzheimer's disease. New Engl J Med 315:485–487

Hyman BT, Van Hoesen GW, Damasio AR, Barnes CL (1984) Alzheimer's disease: cell-specific pathology isolates the hippocampal formation. Science 225:1168–1170

Hyman BT, Van Hoesen GW, Kromer LJ, Damasio AR (1986) Perforant pathway changes and the memory impairment of Alzheimer's disease. Ann Neurol 20:472–481

Lamy C, Duyckaerts C, Delaère P, Payan Ch, Fermanian J, Poulain V, Hauw J-J (1989) Comparison of seven staining methods for senile plaques and neurofibrillary tangles in a prospective series of 15 elderly patients. Neuropathol Appl Neurobiol 15:563–578

Mann DMA (1988) Neuropathological and neurochemical aspects of Alzheimer's disease. In: Iversen LL, Iversen SD, Snyder SH (eds) Handbook of psychopharmacology (vol. 20): Psychopharmacology of the aging nervous system. Plenum Press, New York, pp 1–48

Mesulam M-M (1985) Principles of behavioral neurology. Davis, Philadelphia

Pandya DN, Seltzer B (1982) Association areas of the cerebral cortex. Trends Neurosc 5:386–390

Pearson RC, Esiri MM, Hiorns RW, Wilcock GK, Powell TP (1985) Anatomical correlation of the distribution of the pathological changes in the neocortex in Alzheimer disease. Proc Natl Acad Sci USA 82:4531–4534

Probst A, Basler V, Bron B, Ulrich J (1983) Neuritic plaques in senile dementia of the Alzheimer type: a Golgi analysis in the hippocampal region. Brain Res 268:249–254

Rogers J, Morrison JH (1985) Quantitative morphology and regional and laminar distributions of senile plaques in Alzheimer's disease. J Neurosci 5:2801–2808

Saper CB, German DC, White CL (1985) Neuronal pathology in nucleus basalis and associated cell groups in senile dementia of Alzheimer type: possible role in cell loss. Neurology 35:1089–1095

Saper CB (1988) Chemical neuroanatomy of Alzheimer's disease. In: Iversen LL, Iversen SD, Snyder SH (eds) Handbook of psychopharmacology (vol. 20): Psychopharmacology of the aging nervous system. Plenum Press, New York, pp 131–156

Tagliavini F, Giaccone G, Frangione B, Bugiani O (1988) Preamyloid deposits in the cerebral cortex of patients with Alzheimer's disease and non-demented individuals. Neurosci Lett 93:191–196

Terry RD, Gonatas JK, Weiss M (1964) Ultrastructural studies in Alzheimer presenile dementia. Am J Pathol 44:269–297

Terry RD, Hansen LA, DeTeresa R, Davies P, Tobias H, Katzman R (1987) Senile dementia of the Alzheimer type without neocortical neurofibrillary tangles. J Neuropathol Exp Neurol 46:262–268

Terry RD, Peck A, DeTeresa R, Schechter R, Horoupian DS (1981) Some morphometric aspects of the brain in senile dementia of the Alzheimer type. Ann Neurol 10:184–192

Distribution of Tau-PHF in Brodmann Areas Reveals a Heterogeneity of the Degenerating Process in Rostro-Caudal Regions and as a Function of Age

P. Vermersch, B. Frigard, A. Wattez, and *A. Delacourte*

Summary

Clinical and neuropathological studies have shown evidence of subgroups and heterogeneity in the presentation of Alzheimer's disease (AD). To quantify the degenerating process, we have been able to set up a reliable experimental protocol based upon an immunoblot analysis of pathological tau proteins, referred to as tau 55, 64 and 69, which are known to be early and reliable markers of AD. These markers allowed us to map easily the distribution of the neurofibrillary degeneration. The mapping was performed in the 46 Brodmann areas of the brains from five Alzheimer patients with similar duration of the disease. In all cases, the detection of tau 55, 64 and 69 was positive in all areas except in primary visual cortex (area 17) for two patients. The quantities of abnormal tau were especially strong in temporal neocortical and limbic areas and were higher in associative cortex than in primary sensory cortex. Using this quantitative approach, we observed three factors of heterogeneity:
1. occipital and frontal lobes were sometimes less affected by the degenerating process while limbic and temporal lobes were constantly and strongly affected, showing a heterogenous pattern along the rostrocaudal axis;
2. the comparison of the amounts of abnormal tau proteins found in the temporal area (AB21) of 10 AD patients with different ages of onset was also undertaken. Generally we observed a decrease of the quantity of abnormal tau in late onset cases, but the brain of one very old AD patient contained huge amounts of abnormal tau proteins in all neocortical areas;
3. despite a very short duration of illness (18 months), one patient exhibited a general and large amount of abnormal tau proteins expressed in all cortical areas and in the neostriatum. We conclude that our biochemical approach is very convenient to apprehend the extent and the intensity of the degenerating process. This approach demonstrates the heterogeneity of AD.

Alzheimer's disease (AD) is a neurological disorder characterized by the presence within the central nervous system of extracellular amyloid deposits and intraneuronal neurofibrillary tangles (NFT). Clinical and neuropathological studies have shown evidence of subgroups and heterogeneity in the presentation of the disease (Chui et al., 1986; Mayeux et al., 1985). Some atypical presentations could be linked to a specific distribution of NFT in relation to selectively affected circuits (Hof et al., 1990; Jagust et al., 1990). This distribu-

F. Boller et al. (Eds.)
Heterogeneity of Alzheimer's Disease
© Springer-Verlag Berlin Heidelberg 1992

tion is assessed by histological or immunohistological tools. However, due to technical difficulties, there is a very limited number of reports focusing on a systematic analysis of NFT quantification in the different cortical areas (the 46 Brodmann areas) of AD (Brun and Gustafson, 1976; Arnold et al., 1991) and most investigators have focused their interest on a few selected regions.

The neurofibrillary degeneration in AD consists of the accumulation of paired helical filaments, mainly composed of a triplet of abnormally phosphorylated tau proteins named Tau 55, 64 and 69, or τ PHF (Delacourte et al., 1990; Hanger et al., 1991; Lee et al., 1991). Using these reliable markers, we have elaborated a practical method to quantify the degenerating process in AD and assessed the heterogeneity of the disease as a function of age, duration of the disease and of cortical mapping.

Material and Methods

Eleven patients with neuropathologically confirmed AD were included in the study (Table 1). Five cases had a presenile onset. At autopsy, the left hemisphere was fixed in formalin for neuropathological evaluation and the right hemisphere was dissected at the time of autopsy for biochemical studies. In five cases (cases 1 to 5), tissue samples from cortical areas were dissected by the same investigator (P.V.) using the Brodmann classification (Brodmann, 1909). The identification of Brodmann areas was performed using a standard template atlas (Nieuwenhuys et al., 1988). To avoid inaccuracy in dissection of a few defined regions, the following areas were pooled together: 1 + 3; 2 + 5; 26 + 27 + 30 + 31; 41 + 42. The samples were homogenized in the Laemmli sample buffer 1 : 10 (W/V) and heat-treated (Laemmli, 1970). For immunoblot studies, 20 microliters of each brain homogenate was loaded in a 15-well gel (14–14 cm). Proteins were resolved on 10–20% sodium dodecyl sulfate polyacrylamide gel gradients. They were electrophoretically transferred to nitrocellulose membranes before incubation with the anti-paired helical filaments antibodies

Table 1. Demographic data of the 11 AD patients included in the study

Case	Sex	Type	Age of onset (years)	Age at death (years)	Duration (years)
1	M	Sporadic	69	78	9
2	F	Sporadic	82	90	8
3	F	Sporadic	67	78	11
4	F	Sporadic	65	75	10
5	F	Sporadic	73	82	9
6	M	Sporadic	59	69	10
7	M	Sporadic	58	67	9
8	M	Sporadic	59	64	5
9	M	Familial	41	47	6
10	F	Sporadic	35	39	4
11	F	Sporadic	65	67	2

(PHF; Flament et al., 1989). This anti-PHF was raised against PHF extracted from the frontal cortex of a patient with AD of early onset. This antiserum exclusively labelled the neurofibrillary degeneration at the optical microscopy level and PHF structures at the electron microscopy level (Défossez et al., 1988); on immunoblots, it specifically immunostained abnormal tau proteins (Delacourte and Défossez, 1986; Flament et al., 1989; Delacourte et al., 1990).

For each sample, the immunoblots were measured by densitometry. Blots were digitized on a Macintosh IIx with a ScanJet IIC flatbed scanner (Hewlett Packard) at a resolution of 72 dots per inch, and were saved on an 8-bit gray (256 shades of gray) scale TIFF files. The images of the immunoblots were processed with the public domain program IMAGE 1.35 from W. Rasband (NIH Research Services Branch, NIMH). The areas of the peaks corresponding to tau 55, 64 and 69 detected in the different cortical homogenates were calculated and compared to those of a positive internal standard. This internal standard was from a temporal cortex homogenate from a familial AD case with early onset. It expressed the highest content in abnormal tau proteins among the 100 AD brains examined in our laboratory. The immunodetection intensities for tau 55, 64 and 69 were rated on a scale from 0 (absence of detection) to the arbitrary value of 10 (value of the internal positive standard). The loading of brain samples was adjusted to avoid a saturation of the optical density and to have a linearity between the amount of immunodetected proteins and the quantity of samples. Using 4-chloronaphtol staining, the linearity was obtained with quantities of homogenates up to 20 µl. Usually, each sample was measured at three different concentrations (5, 10 and 20 µl of SDS sample). The scores were reproduced on a cortical map with a 10 levels gray scale. For data analysis, we grouped areas according to lobe, i.e., frontal, parietal, occipital, limbic areas of the temporal lobe and temporal neocortical areas. The intensity of the immunodetection was compared in the temporal area from 10 patients with different ages of onset and in the hippocampus from six patients with a strong difference of disease duration.

Results

First, we verified that the NFT distribution was uniform within each Brodmann area and that it was possible to score the severity of the degenerating process, by analyzing only one sample of each area. Areas 4, 21, 19 and 39 were chosen because they have a large surface of cortex. The quantities of pathological tau proteins (tau 55, 64, 69) immunodetected in different parts from the same Brodmann area were virtually identical, whereas they were different from one Brodmann area to another (Fig. 1). In the five cases where a complete mapping was made (Fig. 2), the detection of tau 55, 64 and 69 was positive in all cortical areas except in area 17 in two patients (Table 2). The detection level was higher in temporal areas implicated in limbic connections, especially areas 34 and 28. The association areas of the neocortex generally had the highest scores of NFT. The detection intensities in area 20, a higher-order visual association cortex of the inferior temporal gyrus, and in visual association areas 18 and 19

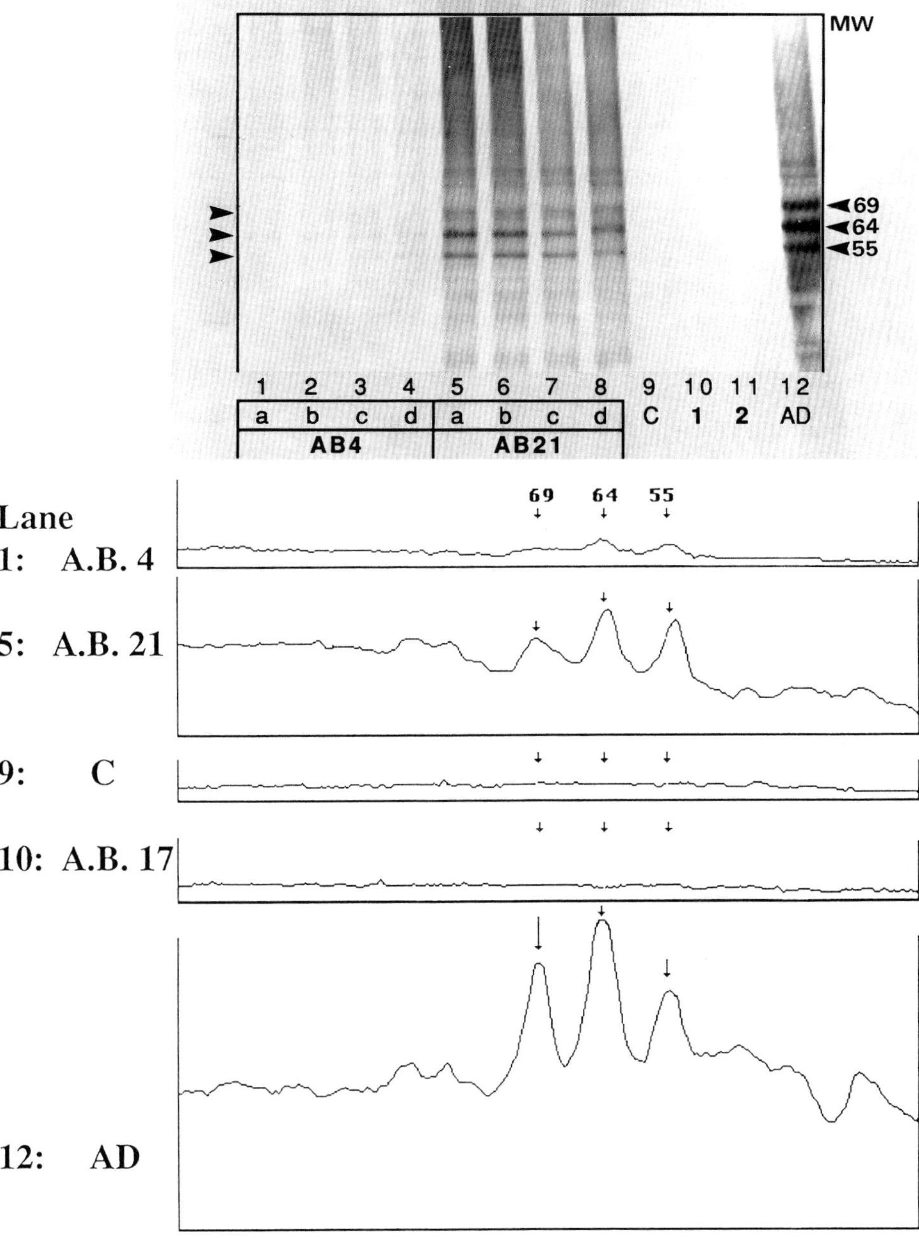

Fig. 1. Immunoblot detection of pathological tau proteins with anti-PHF on brain homogenates from a control and from different AD patients. The scanning of lanes 1, 5, 9, 10, and 12 showed the areas of the peaks corresponding to tau 55, 64 and 69. The blots corresponding to lanes 1, 5, 9, 10, 12 are presented and the triplet of abnormal tau is marked by arrows. There was no detection of tau 55, 64 and 69 in a control subject (lane 9) and in area 17 of case 1 (lane 10) and case 4 (lane 11). The detection seemed relatively equal in four different parts of the same area 4 (AB4) and of the area 21 (AB21) of case 4. Lane 12 corresponds to a brain homogenate from an early onset familial AD case used as an internal positive standard scored 10

Table 2. Scores on a scale of 10 of tau 55, 64 and 69 immunodetection according to Brodmann areas in cases 1 to 5. All areas seemed to be involved in the degenerating process except area 17 in cases 1 and 4. In comparison to the high and relatively equal mean scores in temporal and parietal lobes and in limbic areas, the scores of the frontal and occipital lobes varied considerably between patients

	Case 1	Case 2	Case 3	Case 4	Case 5
Brodman area frontal lobe					
4	5	7	7	1	3
6	2	7	5	5	4
8	1	5	3	4	4
9	7	6	2	7	7
10	1	8	4	7	8
11	3	4	5	5	3
12	3	7	5	5	3
32	5	7	8	6	6
43	4	4	4	2	5
44	1	7	1	5	7
45	4	4	2	6	7
46	3	8	2	6	5
47	3	8	3	5	4
mean scores	3.2 ± 1.7	6.3 ± 1.5	4.1 ± 2.2	4.9 ± 1.7	5.1 ± 1.7
temporal lobe					
20	9	9	9	8	8
21	7	9	8	9	9
22	8	7	8	8	7
36	8	7	7	7	10
37	9	5	4	7	7
41 and 42	4	4	6	3	5
mean scores	7.5 ± 1.8	6.8 ± 2	7 ± 1.7	7 ± 2	7.6 ± 1.7
limbic areas					
23	3	3	5	7	3
24	4	4	4	5	3
25	4	4	5	6	3
26, 27, 29 and 30	2	4	7	6	3
28	10	8	8	9	9
34	9	8	10	9	7
35	7	6	7	6	10
38	9	9	7	7	9
mean scores	6 ± 3.1	5.8 ± 2.3	6.6 ± 1.9	6.8 ± 1.4	5.4 ± 3.1
parietal lobe					
1 and 3	3	6	2	5	1
2 and 5	1	3	3	2	3
7	6	3	3	3	8
31	6	4	5	3	6
39	8	5	9	4	5
40	9	4	8	3	5
mean scores	5.5 ± 3	4.1 ± 1.1	5 ± 2.8	3.3 ± 1	4.6 ± 2.4
occipital lobe					
17	0	3	2	0	2
18	7	9	4	2	4
19	7	7	6	3	7
mean scores	4.6 ± 4	6.3 ± 3	4 ± 2	1.6 ± 1.5	4.3 ± 2.5

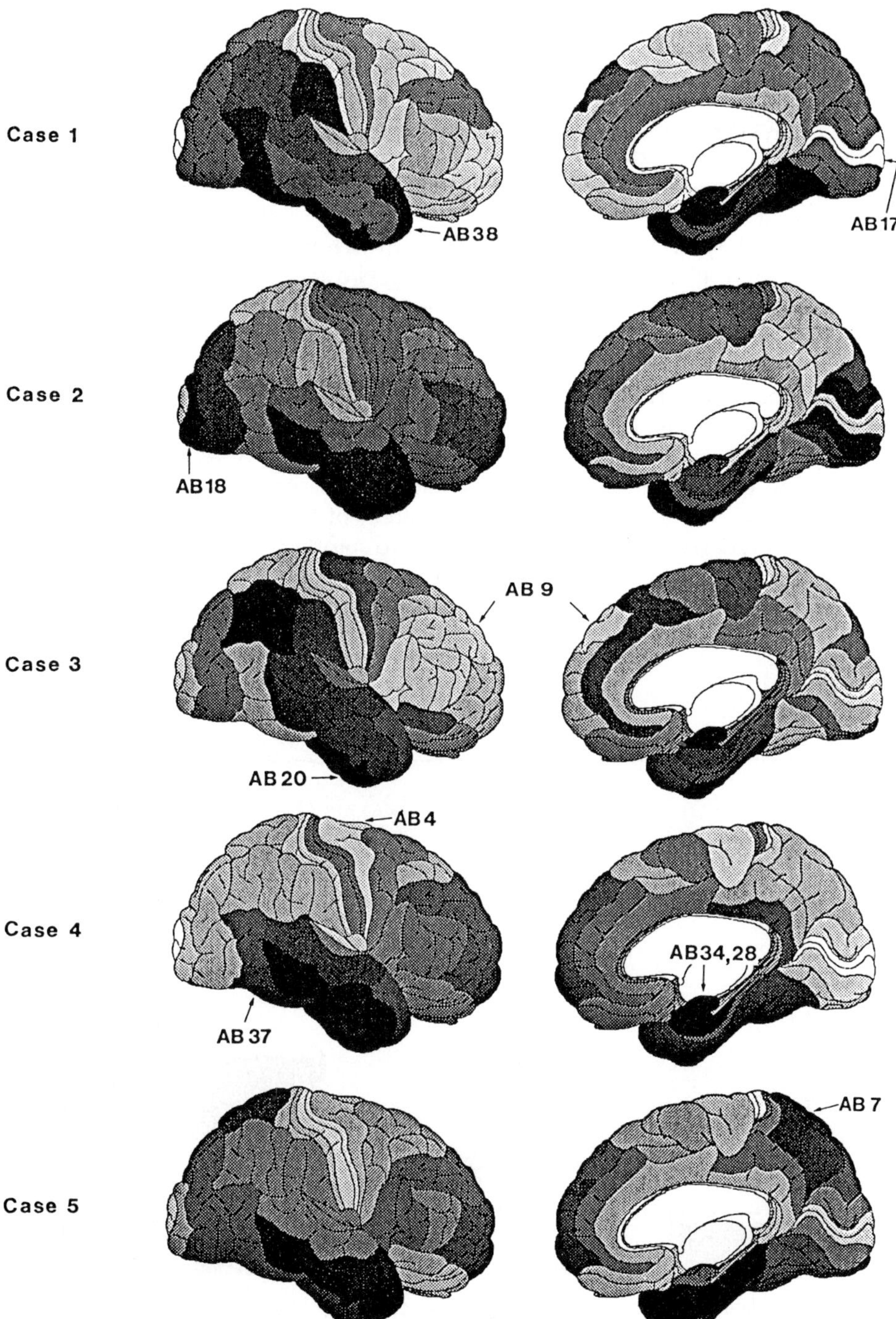

Fig. 2. Mapping of the abnormal tau proteins in 36 Brodmann areas (AB) of five AD patients. The quantity of abnormal tau proteins is represented as a gray scale from 0 (absence of detection) to 10 (very high contentration of abnormal tau). Note that in case 2, the distribution of abnormal tau proteins was present in all cortical areas and that area 17 was spared in case 1 and 4

were higher than in primary visual area 17. In all patients, the detection levels were less pronounced in area 41, the primary auditory region in the Heschl's gyri, than in the portion of area 22 corresponding to the auditory association cortex located immediately lateral to Heschl's gyri in the superior temporal gyrus. In two cases (4 and 5), the score of premotor cortex of area 6 was higher than in primary motor area 4, opposite scores were obtained in two other cases (1 and 3), equal scores in one (case 2). The scores of the parietal lobes were intermediate despite the relatively severe involvement of area 39 (angular gyrus) and area 40 (supramarginal gyrus) in two cases (cases 1 and 3). The mean scores of limbic "lobe" (composed of areas 28, 34, 38, 35, parts of 23 and 24) and temporal lobe (composed of areas 20, 21, 22, 36, 37, 41 and 42) were the highest and relatively equal in the five cases (Table 2). The scores of the posterior cingulate cortex (part of area 23) and of area 24 were lower in the five cases than scores in the other areas of the limbic lobe. Parietal lobe (areas 1, 2, 3, 5, 7, 31, 39 and 40) was intermediate in score, despite relatively high detection in areas 39 and 40 in case 1 and 3. The scores of some prefrontal areas (9, 10, 45, 46) and of the associative areas of the occipital lobe (areas 18 and 19) differed strongly from one patient to another. In comparison to the uniform degree of severe involvement in the limbic and temporal neocortical lobes among patients (mean scores: 6.1 and 7.1; variances: 0.3 and 0.1, respectively), the scores of the occipital (composed of areas 17, 18 and 19) and frontal

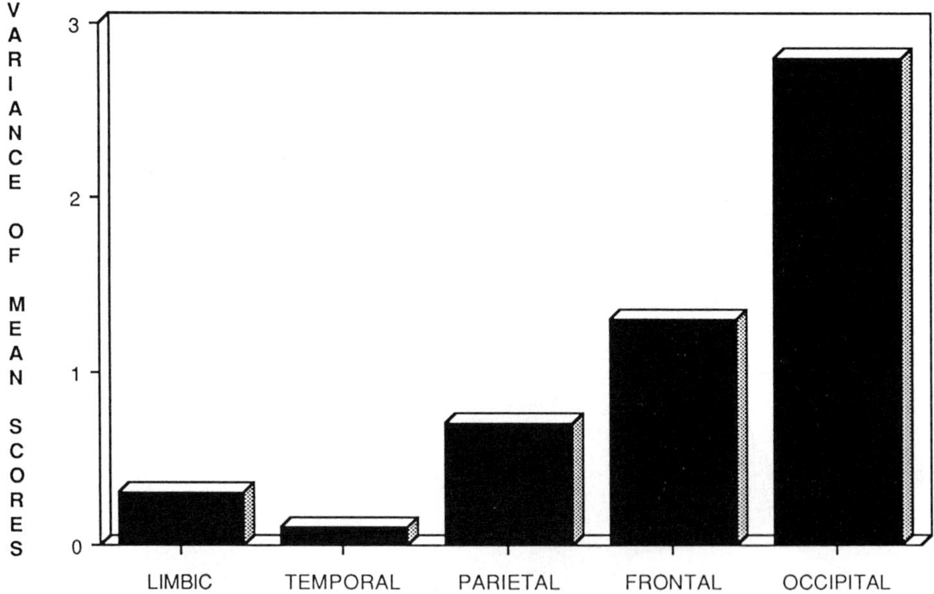

Fig. 3. Variances of mean scores according to lobes. Variances were very low in limbic areas, temporal and parietal lobes and high in frontal and occipital lobes. This difference demonstrated the variability of the distribution of NFT among patients, especially in the occipital and frontal lobes

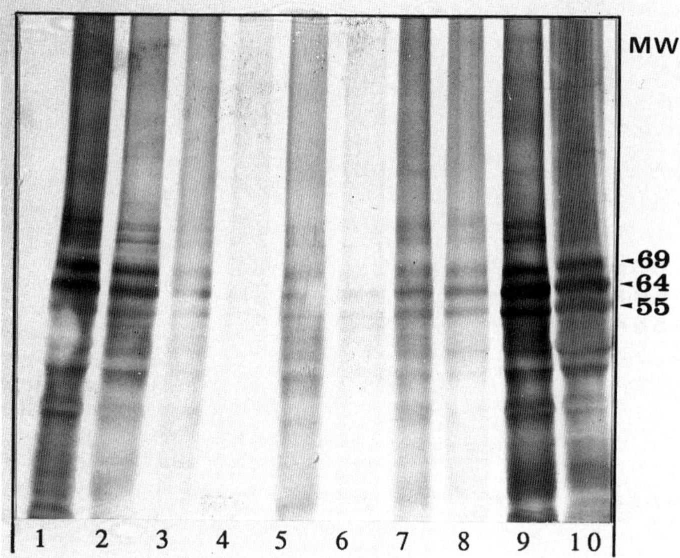

Fig. 4. Comparison of the immunodetection of tau 55, 64 and 69 with a polyclonal antipaired helical filaments antibody in temporal area 21 from 10 AD patients. Except in the patient aged 90 at death (case 2, column 1) and to a lesser degree in case 1, column 2, the immunodetection of abnormal tau proteins is weaker in older patients when compared to the dramatic levels in the youngest cases (9 and 10, columns 9 and 10)

(composed of areas 4, 6, 8, 9, 10, 11, 12, 32, 43, 44, 45, 46, 47) lobes varied considerably between patients, and the variances increased more than 10-fold (mean scores: 4.1 and 4.7; variances: 2.8 and 1.3, respectively; Fig. 3). Variance of mean scores in the parietal lobe also seemed intermediate (0.7).

The comparison of the immunodetection in the temporal cortex of several patients with different ages of onset from 35 to 82 years (Table 1) showed a decreased intensity of immunodetection in late onset, AD patients, except for case 1 and to a lesser degree for case 2 (Fig. 4). The amount of abnormal tau proteins was extremely important in early onset AD patients (cases 9 and 10) and in the hippocampus and the neostriatum from case 11, despite a short duration of the disease (Fig. 5).

Discussion

Abnormally phosphorylated tau proteins, so-called tau 55, 64 and 69, are reliable and early markers of the degenerative process in AD (Flament et al., 1990). To our knowledge, there are only two exhaustive studies of topographical mapping of AD lesions in the different Brodmann areas (Brun and Gustafson, 1976; Arnold et al., 1991) and no report using a biochemical marker of neurofibrillary degeneration. The quantification presented here was based

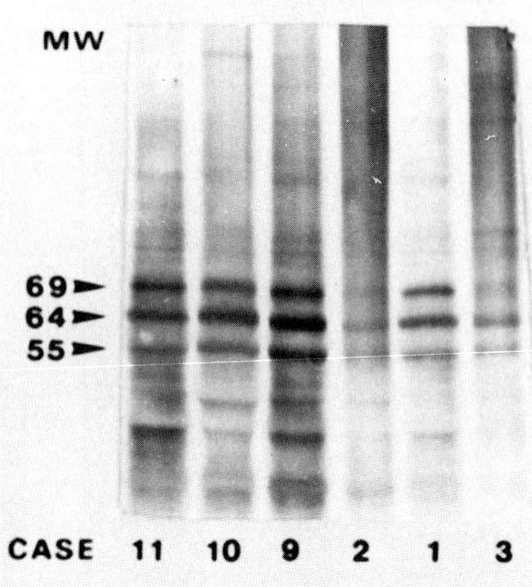

Fig. 5. Comparison of the immunodetection of tau 55, 64 and 69 with a polyclonal antipaired helical filaments antibody in the hippocampus (area 34) from six AD patients with a strong difference in disease duration. Despite a very short disease duration, the immunodetection of the triplet was very strong in cases 11, 10 and 9 and higher than in cases 2, 1 and 3, who had a much longer disease duration

upon a specific detection of the abnormal tau triplet, the basic component of PHF structures, which are found in NFT, in dystrophic neurites of neuritic plaques and in "curly fibers", also referred to as "neuropil thread" (Braak et al., 1986). The triplet corresponds to tau PHF described by other authors (Hanger et al., 1991; Lee et al., 1991). We specifically quantified all the SDS-soluble abnormal tau proteins. Due to the specificity of our antibody and to the fact that Tau 64 and 69 have a molecular weight higher than normal tau, normal tau proteins did not interfere with our quantification (Delacourte et al., 1990). Furthermore, we observed that the triplet is very stable and resists post-mortem delays longer than 24 hours and withstands storage in the deep freeze (below –40°C) for years. Therefore, our biochemical quantification of tau 55, 64 and 69 probably reflects with good accuracy the quantification of PHF structures. Indeed, we found a good correlation between the distribution of tau 55, 64 and 69 and NFT distribution and good parallels between the purification of PHF and the enrichment in abnormal tau proteins (Hanger et al., 1991; Lee et al., 1991; our unpublished results). In principle, it may differe slightly from the distribution of NFT as visualized by thioflavine, which corresponds to "old" NFT possessing the physical properties of the amyloid substance, the young NFT being only labelled with anti-tau or anti-PHF antibodies (Défossez et al., 1988; Schmidt et al., 1988).

Heterogeneity according to the cortical mapping of neurofibrillary degeneration

We confirm that the degenerating process predominates in temporal and associative areas, but this biochemical approach shows that the degenerating process seems to be more extended than previously reported. As in the study by

Arnold et al. (1991), our results shows that the entorhinal cortex and the associated areas of the limbic system had the lowest case-to-case variances for all of the Brodmann's areas. According to the current observations by clinicians (Chui et al., 1985; Mayeux et al., 1985) heterogeneity in topographical distribution of lesions is obvious, even in the small number of patients in our study. The Arnold et al. (1991) study also exhibited strong differences in NFT distribution among patients, but their patient's ages ranged from 63 to 88 at death and duration of illness ranged from 3 to 15 years. Despite the relative clinical homogeneity of the population where our mapping was performed (onset after 65, no case with focal symptoms, similar disease duration, advanced stage of the disease), the intensity of the detection of the abnormal tau triplet differed strongly and major differences appeared in the rostrocaudal distribution. In one case, the maximal detection levels were predominantly located in the posterior areas whereas, in another, the "frontal" areas were more involved.

Heterogeneity as a function of age

In the patient who was oldest (case 2) but who did not have the longest duration of the disease, the detection was relatively high in all cortical areas, including the primary motor and sensory regions. The abnormal tau triplet was found in large amounts in all the cortical areas, demonstrating the general and dramatic involvement of the degenerating process in this very old case of AD with late onset. The intensity of the immunodetection in the temporal cortex (BA 21) was higher than in some younger cases. However, the presenile cases contained very high concentrations of abnormal tau. Previous reports suggested that a more virulent disease process is associated with an earlier onset of AD (Mann et al., 1984; Bondareff, 1983). On neuropathological examination, presenile onset patients manifest greater densities of senile plaques, NFT, cell loss, and choline acetyltransferase depletion (Constantidinis, 1978; Whitehouse et al., 1983; Bird et al., 1983). Quantitative differences in the typical pathology and biochemical markers of AD are also found in patients with a familial history of dementia, or who show myoclonus (Bondareff, 1983; Whitehouse et al., 1983). However, in terms of prediction of course and severity of the disease, there is little consensus about the influence of age of onset. Some extensive studies have shown that in numerous cases of late onset AD, the degenerating process was exclusively found in the hippocampus (Ball et al., 1985; Terry et al., 1987). Cases of old-age demented individuals exhibited abundant cortical amyloid deposits, but neurofibrillary changes were localized exclusively in the entorhinal region; neither Ammon's horn nor isocortex revealed sufficient large numbers of tangles to permit the diagnosis of fully developed AD (Braak and Braak, 1990). Case 2 contrasts dramatically with these data and argues for the heterogeneity of the disease. Despite a very late onset, the cortical involvement was general. Our report shows that the degenerating process could also be severe in late onset AD.

Heterogeneity as a function of the duration of the disease

One of our patients had a rapidly progressive dementia with the typical bio-chemical and neuropathological findings of AD (case 11). The abnormal tau triplet was found in large amounts in all the cortical areas and in the neostriatum. Despite this short duration, the extent of the degenerating process was equal or superior to other cases with a longer disease duration. This result provides biochemical evidence that the disease may be more virulent in some cases, even in sporadic and late onset cases, and therefore also argues for heterogeneity of the disease process.

References

Arnold SE, Hyman BT, Flory J, Damasio AR, Van Hoesen GW (1991) The topographical and neuroanatomical distribution of neurofibrillary tangles and neuritic plaques in the cerebral cortex of patients with Alzheimer's disease. Cerebral Cortex 1:103–116

Ball MJ, Fisman M, Hachinski V, Blume W, Fox A, Kral VA, Kirshen AJ, Fox H (1985) A new definition of Alzheimer's disease: a hippocampal dementia. Lancet i::14–16

Bird TD, Stranahan S, Sumi SM, Raskind M (1983) Alzheimer's disease: choline acetyltransferase activity in brain tissue from clinical and pathological subgroups. Ann Neurol 14:284–293

Bondareff W (1983) Age and Alzheimer disease. Lancet i:1447

Braak H, Braak E, Grundke-Iqbal I, Iqbal K (1986) Occurrence of neuropils threads in the senile human brain and in Alzheimer's disease. A third location of paired helical filaments outside of neurofibrillary tangles and neuritic plaques. Neurosci Lett 65:351–355

Braak H, Braak E (1990) Neurofibrillary changes confined to the entorhinal region and an abundance of cortical amyloid in cases of presenile and senile dementia. Acta Neuropathol 80:479–486

Brodmann K (1909) Vergleichende Lokalisationslehre der Großhirnrinde in ihren Prinzipien dargestellt auf Grund des Zellenbaues. J A Barth, Leipzig, p 324

Brun A, Gustafson L (1976) Distribution of cerebral degeneration in Alzheimer's disease. Arch Psychiat Nervenk 223:15–33

Chui HC, Teng EL, Henderson VW, Moy AC (1985) Clinical subtypes of dementia of the Alzheimer's type. Neurology 35:1544–1550

Constantinidis J (1978) Is Alzheimer's disease a major form of senile dementia? Clinical, anatomical and genetic data. In: Katzman R, Terry RD, Bick KL (eds) Alzheimer's disease, senile dementia and related disorders. Raven, New York, pp 15–25

Défossez A, Beauvillain JC, Delacourte A, Mazzuca M (1988) Alzheimer's disease: a new evidence for common epitopes between microtubule associated protein tau and paired helical filaments (PHF): Demonstration at the electron microscope by a double immuno-gold labelling. Virchows Arch 413:141–145

Delacourte A, Défossez A (1986) Alzheimer's disease: tau proteins, the promoting factors of microtubule assembly, are major components of paired helical filaments. J Neurol Sci 76:173–186

Delacourte A, Flament S, Dibe EM, Hublau P, Sablonnière B, Hémon B, Scherrer V, Défossez A (1990) Pathological Proteins Tau 64 and 69 are specifically expressed in the somatodendritic domain of the degenerating cortical neurons during Alzheimer's disease. Demonstration with a panel of antibodies against Tau proteins. Acta Neuropathol 80:111–117

Flament S, Delacourte A, Hemon B, Défossez A (1989) Characterization of two pathological tau protein variants in Alzheimer brain cortices. J Neurol Sci 92:133–141

Flament S, Delacourte A, Delaère P, Duyckaerts C, Hauw JJ (1990) Correlation between microscopical changes and tau 64 and 69 biochemical detection in senile dementia of the

Hanger DP, Brion JP, Gallo JM, Cairns NJ, Luthert PJ, Anderton BH (1991) Tau in Alzheimer's disease and Down's syndrome is insoluble and abnormally phospharylated. Biochem J 275:99–104

Hof PR, Bouras C, Constantinidis J, Morrison JH (1990) Selective disconnection of specific visual association pathways in cases of Alzheimer's disease presenting with Balint's syndrome. J Neuropathol Exp Neurol 49:168–189

Jagust WJ, Davies P, Tiller-Borcich JK, Reed BR (1990) Focal Alzheimer's disease. Neurology 40:14–19

Laemmli UK (1970) Cleavage of structural proteins during head assembly of bacteriophage T4. Nature 227:680–685

Lee VMY, Balin BJ, Otvos L, Trojanowski JQ (1991) A68: A major subunit of paired helical filaments and derivatized forms of normal Tau. Science 251:675–678

Mann DA, Yates PO, Marcynuik B (1984) Age and Alzheimer's disease. Lancet i:281–282

Mayeux R, Stern Y, Spanton S (1985) Heterogeneity in dementia of the Alzheimer type: evidence of subgroups. Neurology 35:453–461

Nieuwenhuys R, Voogd J, Van Huijzen C (1988) The human central nervous system. A synopsis and atlas. Third Edition Revised. Springer-Verlag, Berlin Heidelberg New York

Schmidt ML, Gur RE, Gur RC, Trojanowski JQ (1988) Intraneuronal and extracellular neurofibrillary tangles exhibit mutually exclusive cytoskeletal antigens. Ann Neurol 23:184–189

Terry RD, Hansen LA, DeTeresa R, Davies P, Tobias H, Katzman R (1987) Senile dementia of the Alzheimer type without neocortical neurofibrillary tangles. J Neuropathol Exp Neurol 46:262–268

Whitehouse PJ, Hedreen JC, White CL, Clark AW, Price DL (1983) Neuronal loss in the basal forebrain cholinergic system in more marked in Alzheimer's disease than in senile dementia of the Alzheimer type. Ann Neurol 14:149

Alzheimer's Disease and Age-Related Pathology in Diffuse Lewy Body Disease

D. W. Dickson, E. Wu, H. A. Crystal, L. A. Matthiace,
S.-H. C. Yen, and P. Davies

Summary

We examined 78 brains with widespread cortical Lewy bodies (mean age: 76.5 ± 9.2). About half of the cases (N = 37) had sufficient neocortical senile plaques (SP) and neurofibrillary tangles (NFT) to warrant a diagnosis of AD. The other half (N = 41) had either few or no SP and no NFT. Concomitant evaluation of 90 brains from participants in prospective clinical studies of aging and dementia (mean age: 83.1 ± 9.0) provided insight into the significance of age-related histopathological lesions. Nondemented old people fell into two distinct pathological groups that were not clinically distinguishable, even with detailed, longitudinal information. One group, which we refer to as pathological aging, had cerebral amyloid deposits sufficient to consider a diagnosis of AD, and the other group, which we refer to as normal aging, had very little or no cerebral amyloid deposits.

Although SP were present in pathological aging, they were diffuse amyloid deposits with either no neuritic elements or dystrophic neurites immunoreactive with anti-ubiquitin, but not Ab39 or Alz50. This distinguished SP in aging from those in AD, which contained Ab39- and Alz50-immunoreactive, thioflavin-S fluorescent neurites. AD brains also invariably had neocortical NFT and neuropil threads, neurofibrillary degeneration in the hippocampus, amygdala and basal forebrain, and amyloid angiopathy. Amyloid angiopathy was present in less than half of the nondemented control brains. In diffuse Lewy body disease (DLBD) the frequency of amyloid angiopathy reflected the extent of co-existing AD. Thus, Alzheimer-type pathology in DLBD cases overlapped with normal aging, pathological aging or AD. In addition, DLBD cases had ubiquitin-immunoreactive neuritic degeneration in the CA2/3 region of the hippocampus not seen in aging or AD. The results suggest that DLBD is a distinct disease that can occur in independent of or co-existent with pathological aging or AD.

Introduction

Diffuse Lewy body disease (DLBD) is a primary degenerative dementia (Burkhardt et al., 1988; Byrne et al., 1988; Crystal et al., 1990; Dickson et al., 1987; Gibb et al., 1987; Hansen et al., 1990; Kosaka et al., 1984; Perry et al., 1990)

F. Boller et al. (Eds.)
Heterogeneity of Alzheimer's Disease
© Springer-Verlag Berlin Heidelberg 1992

characterized by widespread intraneuronal inclusions that have similar antigenic (Bancher et al., 1989; Dickson et al., 1985; Galloway et al., 1988; Goldman et al., 1983; Kuzuhara et al., 1988; Lowe et al., 1988; Pappolla et al., 1986; Schmidt et al., 1991; Wisniewski et al., 1991) and structural features (Forno, 1986; Dickson et al., 1989; Pappolla, 1986) to Lewy bodies of idiopathic Parkinson's disease. In the cerebrum, so-called cortical Lewy bodies (cLB) are most common in lower layers of the limbic and insular cortices. They are also common in the amygdala. A small number of cLB are present in limbic cortices in idiopathic Parkinson's disease (Jellinger, 1989), but they are more numerous and widespread in DLBD.

A common nomenclature for this disorder does not currently exist, and it is variously referred to as Lewy body dementia (Gibb et al., 1989), diffuse Lewy body disease (Kosaka et al., 1985), senile dementia of the Lewy body type (Perry et al., 1989) and Lewy body variant of Alzheimer's disease (Hansen et al., 1990). Although some investigators would restrict the term DLBD to cases with very many cLB, qualitative differences between this form of the disease and cases with fewer, but still widespread, cLB do not exist, and we agree with the school of thought that considers DLBD to be a spectrum of disorders associated with cLB (Kosaka et al., 1983; Dickson et al., 1990a).

Cortical Lewy bodies are round to slightly irregular cytoplasmic inclusions in small nonpyramidal neurons in cortical layers 5 and 6, while neurofibrillary tangles (NFT) are filamentous inclusions in pyramidal neurons of layers 3 and 5. Although cLB can be seen with the hematoxylin and eosin stain, the most sensitive method for detecting cLB is ubiquitin immunocytochemistry (Lennox et al., 1989). Ubiquitin is a 76 amino acid highly conserved protein that is involved in protein folding and nonlysosomal proteolytic degradation of denatured or otherwise abnormal proteins (Finley and Varshavsky, 1985). Ubiquitin has been detected in a wide variety of cellular inclusions, many, but not all, of which are composed of filamentous proteins, such as NFT and Lewy bodies (Lowe et al., 1988). Double immunostaining of sections with antibodies to ubiquitin and NFT is a useful adjunct in the diagnostic evaluation of DLBD cases in which both types of lesions are present (Dickson et al., 1989).

Many cases of DLBD, especially patients older than 60 years of age, have cortical senile plaques (SP). This finding has lead to controversy as to whether DLBD is a variant of AD (Hansen et al., 1990) or a separate disease entity (Dickson, 1990). A consistent finding in pathological studies of DLBD is neuronal loss in brainstem and diencephalic nuclei that are also affected in idiopathic Parkinson's disease, including the substantia nigra and the basal nucleus of Meynert (nbM). Substantial neuronal loss in the substantia nigra is not, however, characteristic of AD. Since the nbM is the major source of cholinergic innervation of the cerebral cortex (Richardson and DeLong, 1988), it is not surprising that cholinergic deficits have been demonstrated in the cerebral cortex in DLBD (Dickson et al., 1987; Hansen et al., 1990; Perry et al., 1990). Intrinsic cortical neurotransmitter (e.g., somatostatin) deficits have also been reported (Dickson et al., 1987; Hansen et al., 1990). Dopaminergic deficits in the basal ganglia similar to those seen in Parkinson's disease have also been described (Perry et al., 1990).

Hippocampal pathology, which is an invariant feature of AD (Ball et al., 1986), is absent in a substantial number of cases of DLBD (Dickson et al., 1989, 1991; Gibb et al., 1989; Ince et al., 1991). The paucity of hippocampal pathology in DLBD is reflected in neurochemical findings. Whereas cortical cholinergic abnormalities are the rule in DLBD, such deficits are inconsistent in the hippocampus; this differentiates DLBD from AD, where hippocampal cholinergic activity is consistently reduced (Davies, 1979). The hippocampus is a primary location for neurofibrillary degeneration AD. The CA-1 region of Ammon's horn and the subiculum appear to be particularly vulnerable (Hirano and Zimmerman, 1962). In contrast, the CA-1 and subicular regions are usually spared in DLBD. On the other hand, neuritic degeneration is very common in CA2/3 in DLBD (Dickson et al., 1991). Neurites with an immunoreactivity profile similar to those in the CA2/3 region of the hippocampus are also found in other regions of the brain in DLBD, including the basal forebrain, substantia nigra, pedunculopontine nuclei, raphe nuclei and dorsal motor nuclei of the vagus (unpublished observations).

The clinical manifestations of DLBD are heterogeneous. In general, early onset cases tend to present with Parkinsonism that may be atypical in its response to levodopa or other clinical features (Kosaka et al., 1988; Kosaka, 1990; Mark et al., 1992; Yoshimura et al., 1988). On the other hand, late onset cases usually have cognitive decline that overshadows extra-pyramidal motor deficits (Burkhardt et al., 1988; Byrne et al., 1989; Crystal et al., 1990; Gibb et al., 1987; Kosaka, 1990; Jellinger et al., 1990; Perry et al., 1990), and such individuals usually come to autopsy with a diagnosis of AD. In several recent autopsy series, DLBD has been recognized as the second most common form of degenerative dementia (7–30%) after AD (Dickson et al., 1989; Hansen et al., 1990; Lennox et al., 1989).

The purpose of this report is to review the neuropathological features of a series of 78 cases of DLBD and consider the evidence for and against it being a variant of AD.

Materials and Methods

Case material

Neuropathologic findings in 78 consecutive cases of DLBD, either autopsied at or referred to the Diagnostic Neuropathology Service at Albert Einstein College of Medicine, are described. For some analyses, DLBD cases were further divided into two groups according to the presence of coexistent AD (DLBD/AD) or absence of AD (pure DLBD; pDLBD). The pathological definition of AD (Khachaturian, 1985) is currently undergoing reappraisal due in part to reports of nondemented elderly subjects with numerous senile plaques sufficient to warrant a diagnosis of AD (Crystal et al., 1988; Delaere et al., 1990; Dickson et al., 1992; Katzman et al., 1988). In this study, a pathological diagnosis of AD required the presence of neocortical NFT and neuropil threads (Braak et al., 1986), and is similar to the criteria proposed by Tomlinson (1989). The DLBD cases were compared to 34 normal elderly controls who had no documented history of dementia and included some subjects from the Bronx Aging Study (Katzman et al., 1989), as well as 34 recent AD cases with no evidence of Lewy bodies in the brainstem or cortex.

Neuropathologic methods

All brains were evaluated with thioflavin-S fluorescent microscopy. Thioflavin-S is a very sensitive method for detecting cerebral amyloid (Schwartz 1970). SP were also counted in 10x fields from at least five cortical sections as previously described (Dickson et al., 1992). NFT were counted in 40x fields. The results reflect an average of three fields. NFT were counted in layers 3 to 5 to maximize the number of lesions. Cortical Lewy bodies were counted in 10x fields from the parahippocampal gyrus using ubiquitin-stained sections or double immunostained sections when NFT were also present.

Immunocytochemistry

Immunocytochemical studies were performed on paraffin sections in all cases and on vibratome sections in a subset of cases. All cases were studied with ubiquitin immunocytochemistry using previously published methods and a rabbit polyclonal antibody to ubiquitin (Dickson et al., 1990b). Other antibodies used to evaluate the cases included an affinity-purified antibody to a synthetic peptide with the sequence of the first 25 amino acids of $\beta/A4$ (Dickson et al., 1989), as well as monoclonal antibodies to NFT (Ab39; Yen et al., 1987) and Alz-50 (Wolozin et al., 1986). Double immunostaining was performed using a procedure previously described in our laboratory (Kure et al., 1990).

Results

Clinical features

The breakdown of the cases included 41 pDLBD and 37 DLBD/AD. The average age at the time of death was 73.7 ± 9.8 years for pDLBD and 79.8 ± 6.9 years for DLBD/AD. The male to female ratio for pDLBD was $31:6$ (76% men) and, for DLBD/AD, $23:14$ (62% men). In contrast, the ratio for the 34 consecutive AD cases was $10:34$ (71% women; average age, 80.8 ± 7.2 years). The male predominance of DLBD noted in our original series of cases (Dickson et al., 1989) has continued to hold true in the larger series. Although not specifically emphasized in other reports, more men than women have been reported with DLBD. These results are interesting in light of increasing evidence for sexual differences in the differentiation of monoaminergic neurons (Reisert and Pilgrim, 1991).

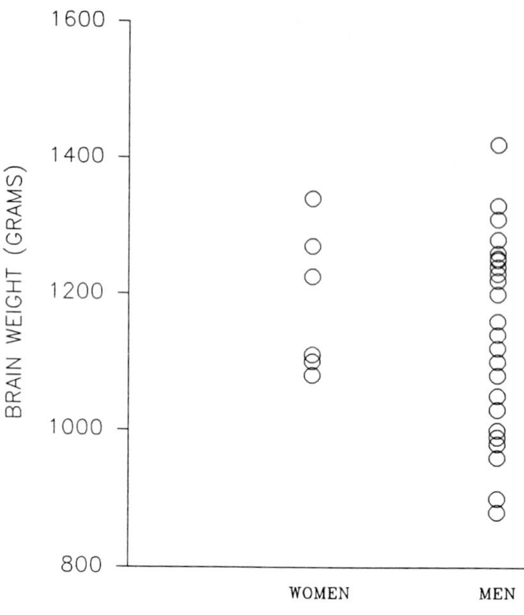

Fig. 1. Brain weights were derived from formalin fixed specimens. In cases where only half the brain was available due to submission of the other half for biochemical studies, the weight was determined by multiplying the weight of one half by 2

Brain weight

The average brain weight for pDLBD was 1263 ± 131 grams and, for DLBD/AD, 1132 ± 139 grams. The average brain weight for AD was significantly smaller, 996 ± 198 grams. The distribution of brain weights for DLBD with respect to sex is shown in Figure 1. The brain weight of DLBD did not differ significantly from nondemented elderly controls (1202 ± 119 grams). Analysis of variance indicated that disease, independent of gender, was responsible for some of the differences observed for brain weights in DLBD compared to AD. A grossly normal brain, except for depigmentation of the substantia nigra, in a man with dementia of sometimes short duration (Armstrong et al., 1991) is a typical presentation for DLBD.

Neocortex

Senile plaques – quantitative aspects

Most DLBD cases in this series had enough SP in the middle frontal gyrus to warrant consideration of a diagnosis of AD. All cases of DLBD/AD met provisional criteria for AD (Khachaturian, 1985), but only 27% of pDLBD cases met these same age-adjusted criteria. The cases that failed to meet the criteria included those that had either no or too few SP, as well as those with sufficient SP, but aged less than 75. AD without NFT is only recognized in individuals greater than 75 years of age in the Khachaturian criteria; however,

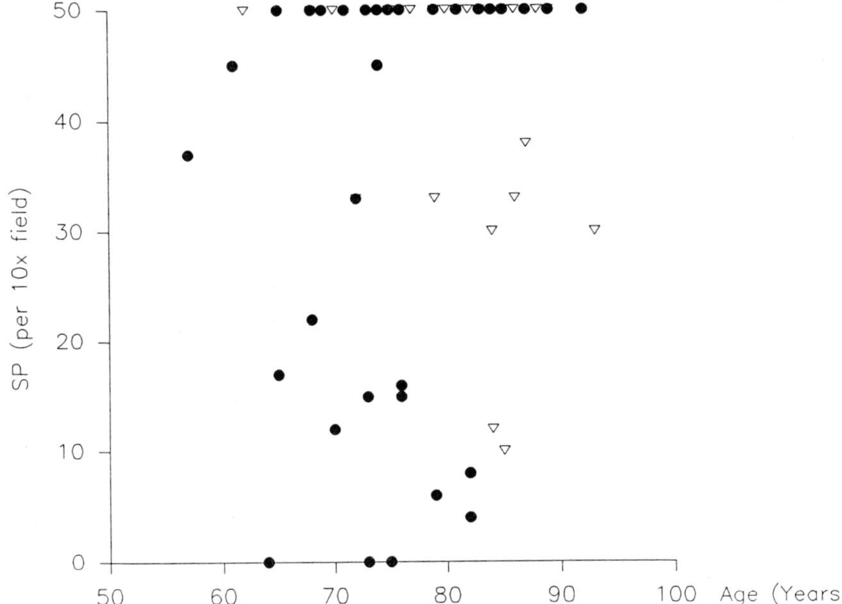

Fig. 2. The average number of senile plaques in a 10x field on thioflavin-S stained sections from the middle frontal gyrus section. The solid circles are cases of pure DLBD and the open inverted triangles are cases of DLBD/AD

if age is not considered, 82% of the DLBD cases had enough SP to consider a diagnosis of AD. The presence of numerous SP in the middle frontal gyrus did not always correlate with a similar extent of SP in other cortical areas, however. This discrepancy has also been noted in pathological aging cases, and it suggests that frontal association cortices may be particularly vulnerable to amyloid deposition.

The number of SP tended to increase with age for pDLBD, although there were several cases with no SP despite an advanced age. On the other hand, an oppositve trend was noted for DLBD/AD, with a decreasing number of SP with increasing age (Fig. 2). Our studies suggested that SP were more common in DLBD than in the elderly controls, and approached the number seen in AD cases when they had co-existing AD (AD, 46.7 ± 7.8; DLBD/AD, 45.1 ± 10.4; pDLBD, 32 ± 20.9; controls, 11 ± 20.5). The variance was greatest for elderly controls and pDLBD because of inclusion of cases with no SP and cases with many SP.

Senile plaques – qualitative aspects

Studies of qualitative differences in SP in AD, DLBD and aging were performed with fluorescent histochemistry and immunocytochemistry. With thiof-

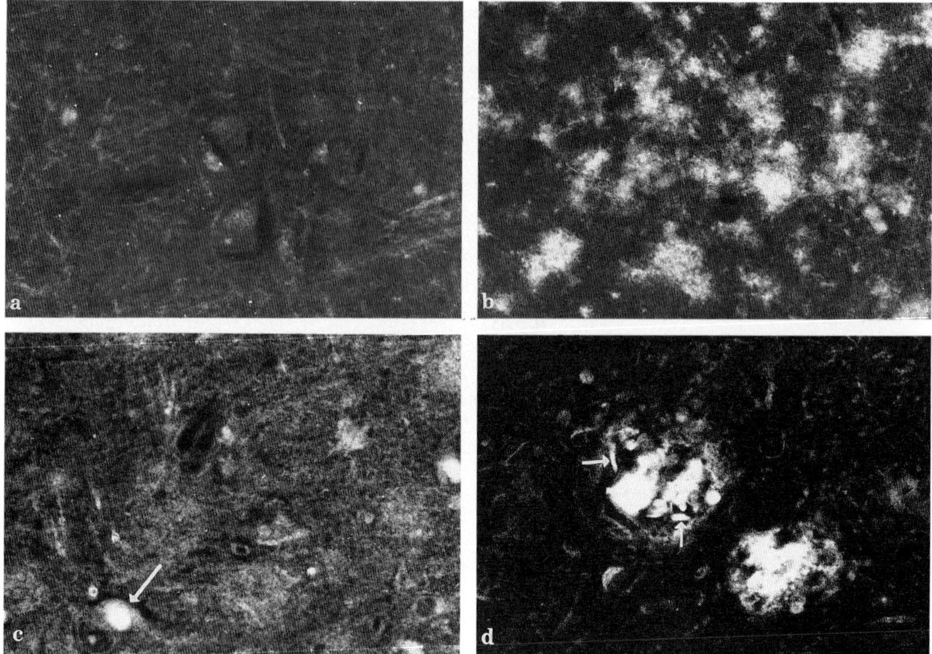

Fig. 3a–d. Thioflavin-S stained sections from normal aging (*a*), pathological aging (*b*), DLBD (*c*) and AD (*d*). The SP in both pathological aging and DLBD are diffuse amyloid deposits, without fluorescent neurites as in SP of AD (arrows in d). Arrow in c indicates a cortical Lewy body

lavin-S stains, nondemented elderly controls fell into two groups: those with no or very few SP (normal aging; Fig. 3a) and those with numerous SP (pathological; Fig. 3b). In pathological aging, SP were almost all diffuse amyloid deposits few or no neuritic components. Senile plaques in pDLBD were similar to those in pathological aging (Fig. 3c). Many of SP in AD and in DLBD/AD differed by the presence of fluorescent curvilinear profiles (Fig. 3d). Double-labeling and ultrastructural studies show that these profiles corresponded to neurites with paired helical filaments (PHF). It is, of course, also true that diffuse SP are common in AD, and they are the predominant form of SP in the cerebellar cortex (Dickson et al., 1990c), whereas incidentally, SP are rarely found in pathological aging and DLBD (unpublished observation).

With immunocytochemistry, the SP of pathological aging, DLBD and AD all contained β/A4 immunoreactive deposits. Although most diffuse SP are little more than amyloid deposits without apparent disturbance of the neuropil (Masliah et al., 1990), those amyloid deposits with more compact amyloid cores often were surrounded by ubiquitin-immunoreactive granular dystrophic neurites (Fig. 4; Dickson et al., 1989, 1990b). In pDLBD and pathological aging diffuse SP and SP with compact amyloid cores in the cerebral cortex lacked neurites stained with antibodies to NFT (Ab39) or Alz-50. Exceptions to this rule were sometimes found in the few SP in the amygdala and subicu-

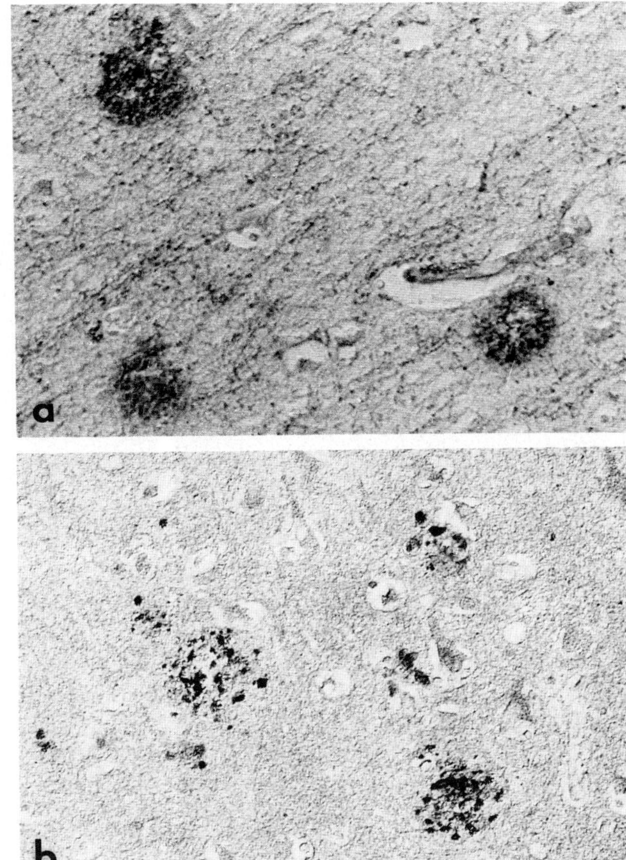

Fig. 4a, b. Immunocyto-chemistry of the cerebral cortex in DLBD with an antibody to β/A4 amyloid reveals diffuse and more compact amyloid deposits (*a*). Some of the SP had granular, round dystrophic neurites with anti-ubiquitin immunostaining (*b*). Similar staining is seen in pathological aging (Dickson et al., 1990, 1992)

lum, where SP sometimes had PHF-type neurites. In the cortices of AD and DLBD/AD, SP were consistently immunostained with Ab39 and Alz-50. In addition, both antibodies stained numerous neuropil threads throughout the cortex, amygdala and hippocampus that were not present in normal or pathological aging or pDLBD.

Neuronal changes

The nature of the neuronal degeneration in DLBD is different from that in AD. The characteristic lesion in cortical neurons in AD is the NFT, while in DLBD it is the cLB. With thioflavin-S fluorescent microscopy NFT are brightly stained, filamentous inclusions, (Fig. 5a), whereas cLB are weakly fluorescent, round inclusions (Fig. 5b). The number of NFT with respect to age for pDLBD and DLBD/AD is shown in Figure 6. None of the pDLBD cases had cortical NFT, by definition. Even in cases with DLBD/AD, the number of midfrontal

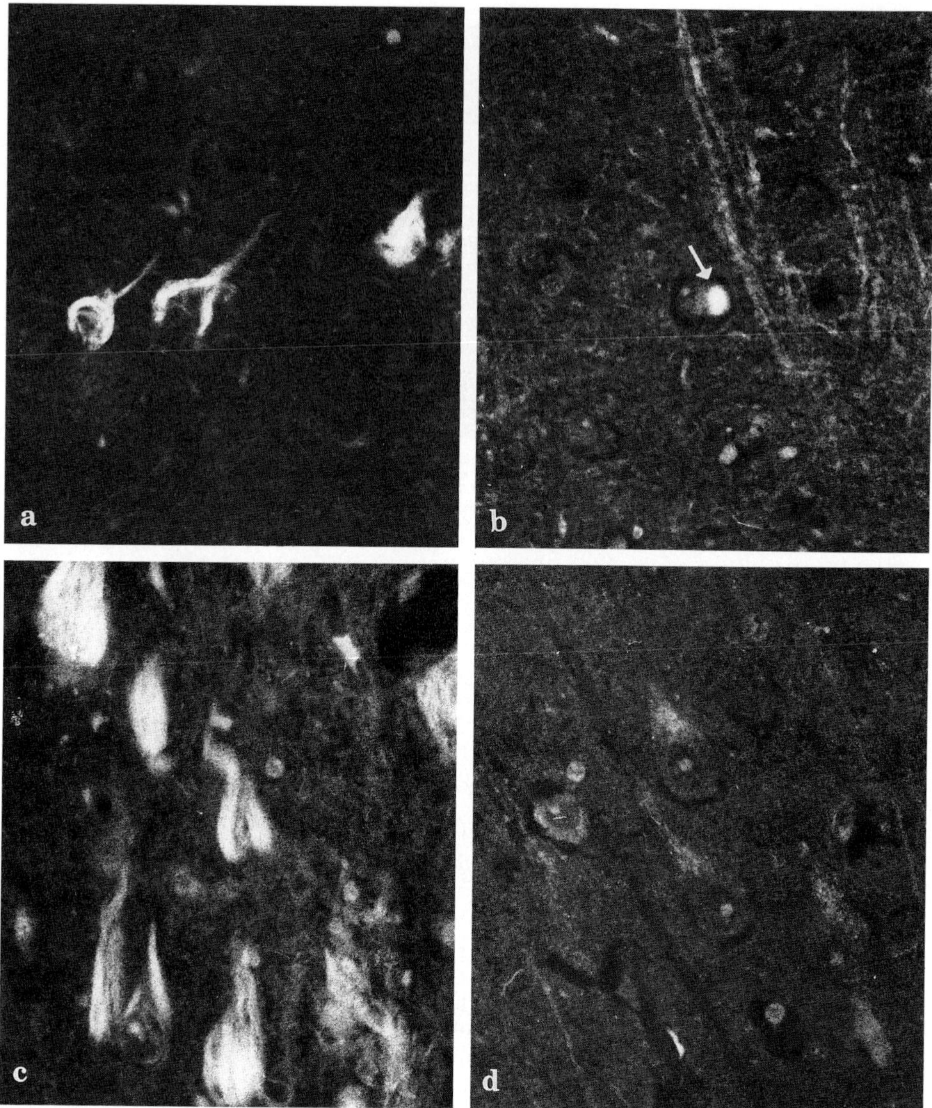

Fig. 5a–d. Cortical neuronal changes in AD are filamentous intraneuronal inclusions, NFT (*a*), while round, weakly fluorescent cLB (arrow) are found in DLBD (*b*). In the hippocampus, AD cases display consistent NFT in CA-1 region (*c*), whereas this area is sometimes devoid of lesions in DLBD (*d*)

gyrus NFT was sparse. Regional studies currently ongoing in our laboratory suggest that the frontal association areas are relatively resistent to neurofibrillary degeneration in AD (unpublished observations). No cLB were detected in AD or nondemented control brains. The average number of cLB in the parahippocampal gyrus was 4.9 ± 6.6 for pDLBD and 2.8 ± 1.9 for DLBD/AD.

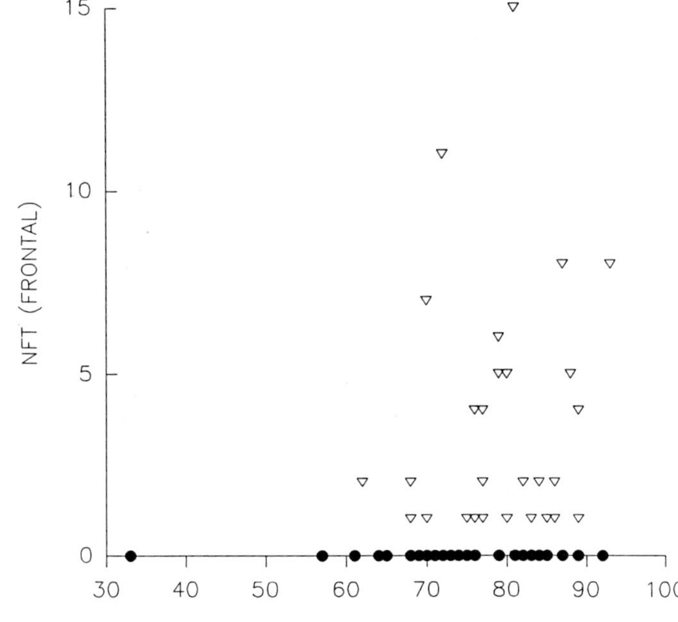

Fig. 6. The number of NFT in the middle frontal gyrus with respect to diagnosis (pDLBD, solid circles; DLBD/AD, open inverted triangles) and age. Each count reflects an average of three 40x fields

Amyloid angiopathy

In a smaller subset of DLBD cases (N = 68), amyloid angiopathy was assessed by rigorous morphometric methods (Wu et al., 1992). Amyloid angiopathy was detected in parenchymal vessels of 97% of AD and 85% of DLBD/AD cases, but only 43% of pDLBD and 38% of nondemented elderly controls (Wu et al., 1992). These results suggest that the frequency of amyloid angiopathy in DLBD reflects processes that are not intrinsic to DLBD, but rather to co-existing AD or pathological aging.

Hippocampus

Neurofibrillary tangles

Hippocampal neurofibrillary degeneration is an invariant manifestation of AD (Ball et al., 1983; Fig. 5c), but this is decidedly not true for DLBD (Dickson et al., 1991; Hansen et al., 1991; Ince et al., 1991). While NFT are usually present in the hippocampus in DLBD/AD in at least small numbers, the hippocampus is spared of NFT (Fig. 5d; Dickson et al., 1989), in approximately half of the cases of pDLBD.

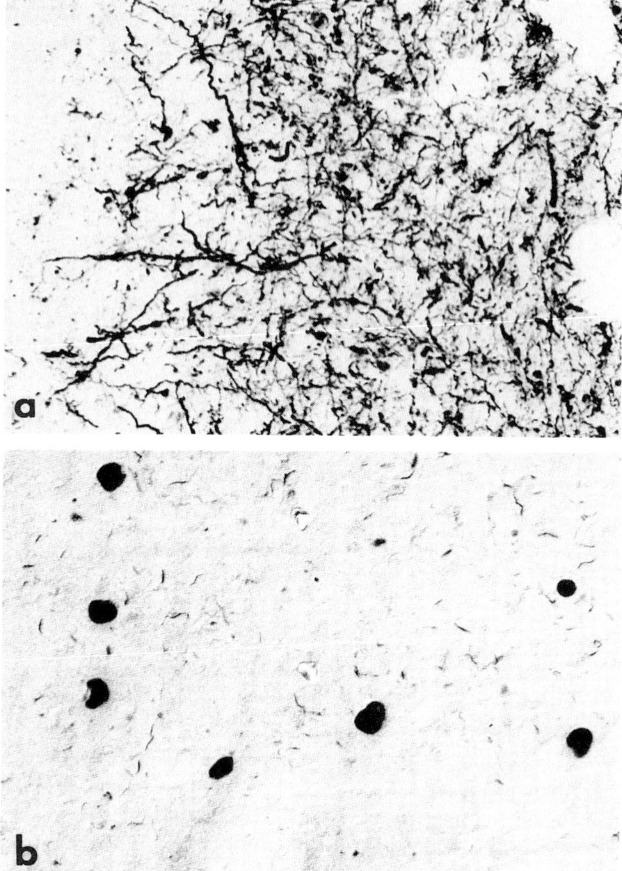

Fig. 7 a, b. Anti-ubiquitin immunocytochemistry of the CA2/3 region of DLBD reveals a dense network of immunoreactive processes (*a*). The adjacent CA1 region had none of this type of neurites, but there were a few NFT. The parahippocampal gyrus from the same case had numerous cortical Lewy bodies in the deeper layers (*b*). A few neuropil threads were also present, but these were not found in the neocortex

Neuritic degeneration

Ubiquitin immunocytochemistry has revealed a type of neuritic degeneration that is highly prevalent in DLBD (Dickson et al., 1991). This DLBD-specific neuritic degeneration was present in the CA2/3 region, a region that is usually spared in AD. The neurites are long, tortuous and sometimes segmented (Fig. 7). They are stained with antibodies to ubiquitin and inconsistently with neurofilament monoclonal antibodies, but even less consistently with Alz-50 and not at all with Ab39. At the electron microscopic level they contain intermediate size filaments (about 10 nm diameter), and they are sometimes detected in myelinated processes. Their immunoreactivity profile was similar to that of cLB; however, in contrast to cLB, which could be seen on H & E stains or thioflavin-S fluorescent microscopy, CA2/3 neurites were not visible with routine histology or thioflavin-S.

In this larger series of cases, the extent of CA2/3 neuritic degeneration correlated with the density of cLB, as previously noted (Dickson et al., 1991).

We have recently encountered sparse CA2/3 neurites in several new cases of idiopathic Parkinson's disease (generously donated by Dr. Josefina Llena, Montefiore Medical Center) that had very sparse cLB. We have not detected them in other degenerative diseases, such as corticobasal ganglionic degeneration, striatonigral degeneration or dementia lacking distinctive histopathology, all of which are disorders with degeneration of substantia nigra.

Basal nucleus of Meynert

The nbM was one of the first areas where Lewy bodies were first described (Gibb and Poewe, 1986). Invariably, there is neuronal loss in the basal nucleus in DLBD (Dickson et al., 1987; Gibb et al., 1989; Perry et al., 1990), and it is often more severe than in AD. Accompanying neuronal loss in the nbM are Lewy bodies in residual neurons and frequently in neuronal processes (Fig. 8). In contrast, NFT are present in almost every case of AD (Fig. 8).

Discussion

Critical to the discussion of the nature of Alzheimer-type pathology in DLBD is a need for criteria for the pathological diagnosis of AD. At present there is no universal agreement as to criteria for AD; neither is it even certain that AD is a single pathological entity (St. George-Hyslop et al., 1990). There is no question that β/A4 amyloid deposits in the brain and cerebral blood vessels (Glenner, 1979) are characteristic of AD, but is AD only β-amyloid deposition? If amyloid deposition is the defining feature of AD, then well over 80% of elderly subjects have AD based upon neuropathologic studies of human brains by several investigative groups (Tomlinson et al., 1976; Davies et al., 1988), as well as clinicopathologic correlations ongoing in our laboratory (Dickson et al., 1992). Since amyloid deposition is a relatively nonspecific phenomenon outside of the central nervous system, it seems reasonable to suggest that cerebral amyloidosis may also be a relatively nonspecific manifestation of a variety of conditions. The list of disorders in which β-amyloid deposition has been described continues to grow. It includes AD, Down's syndrome, pathological aging in both humans and other mammals, dementia pugilistica and following acute head trauma, familial amyloid angiopathies, Guam parkinsonism-dementia complex and other non-Alzheimer dementias (Guiroy et al., 1991; Mann and Jones, 1990; Roberts et al., 1991, 1992; Selkoe et al., 1987).

The neuropathology of AD uniformly includes other features, including neuronal loss in certain brainstem and diencephalic nuclei, hippocampal granulovacuolar degeneration and Hirano body formation, cortical astrocytic gliosis and microglial activation, and diffuse amyloid deposits in the basal ganglia and cerebellar cortex, in addition to cortical, hippocampal and amygdaloid neurofibrillary degeneration. These lesions do not by any means strictly co-localize. Discrete brain regions display specific and predictable vulnerabilites to these lesions in AD. The likelihood that simple overproduction of an amyloidogen-

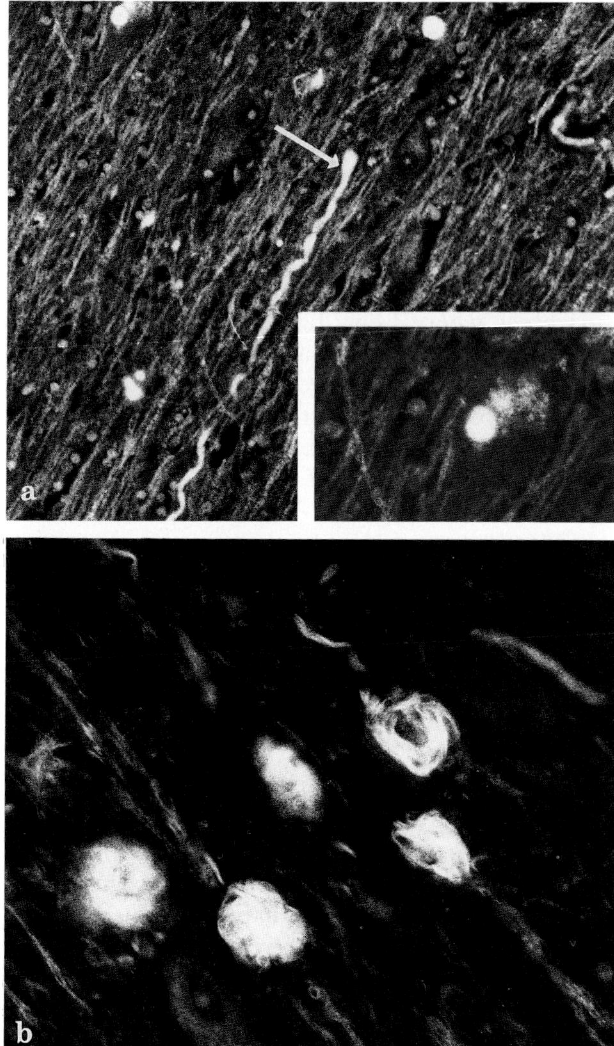

Fig. 8a, b. The basal nucleus of Meynert displays distinctive pathology with thioflavin-S in DLBD (*a*) and AD (*b*). In DLBD, neurons contain Lewy bodies (inset) and some processes contain so-called neuritic Lewy bodies (arrow). In AD, on the other hand, neurons contain globose NFT (b)

etic component of the amyloid precursor protein could lead to this constellation of findings has been further diminished in light of the retraction (Robertson, 1992) of recent reports that transgenic animals expressing excessive amyloid precursor protein develop NFT, neuritic SP and neuropil threads (Kawabata et al., 1991).

While β/A4 amyloid has been detected in a variety of animal species (Selkoe et al., 1987), PHF have not been described in any species other than man. Although NFT are also detected in several non-AD brain diseases, for the most part, these are rare conditions. Furthermore, the extensive alteration of the neocortical neuropil (PHF-containing neuropil threads) in AD are not detected in these other disorders. Using quantitative immunoassay, antibodies that detect tau protein, in particular abnormal forms of tau protein (A68 or PHF-tau), clearly differentiate AD from normals and non-AD dementias (Ghanbari et al., 1990). Our working hypothesis ist that PHF formation in neurons and their processes is the defining feature of AD (Dickson and Yen, 1989). Based upon clinicopathological correlations, PHF and other markers of neuronal injury (e.g., synaptophysin immunoreactivity) display the best correlations with clinical cognitive impairment (Delaere et al., 1989; Dickson et al., 1988; McKee et al., 1991; Terry et al., 1991).

The high frequency of AD in adult Down's syndrome, the location of the amyloid precursor protein gene on chromosome 21 and identification of loci for familial AD on chromosome 21 (Tanzi et al., 1989) provide compelling evidence that β/A4 amyloid is a fundamental component of AD (Hardy and Allsop, 1991). Nevertheless, pathology very similar to AD has also been described in families with mutations in the Prp gene (Ghetti et al., 1989). These features all suggest that amyloid deposition may be necessary, but not sufficient, to produce AD.

Although it is true that chromosome 21 is the chromosome carrying the genetic locus for a few families with AD (Tanzi et al., 1989; Goate et al., 1990), other families have shown linkage to chromosome 19 and still others to non-21, non-19 loci (Schellenberg et al., 1988; Roses et al., 1987; St. George-Hyslop et al., 1990). This finding has prompted some investigators to suggest a multilocus model of AD (Roses et al., 1991). Such a complex model seems reasonable, given the complex nature of the pathology of AD.

What then of Alzheimer-type pathology in DLBD? Is DLBD a variant of AD? This consideration is apparently not reasonable in younger individuals with DLBD who present with Parkinsonism, without cognitive deficits. Such individuals usually have few, if any, changes of the AD type. Complete absence of AD type changes is also characteristic of a minority of late onset cases of DLBD. It is perhaps worth noting that some non-demented elderly humans also have no AD type pathology, but they are a small minority.

Older onset cases of DLBD with either amyloid deposits alone (pDLBD), or amyloid deposits and NFT (DLBD/AD), share a number of pathological features with DLBD cases lacking AD type changes, including degeneration of substantia nigra and nbM, brainstem and cortical Lewy bodies, and CA2/3 neuritic degeneration of the hippocampus. Although some late onset cases have few or no SP, the majority have at least some SP. Given the advanced age of most subjects, it seems likely that amyloid deposition in DLBD represents a manifestation of pathological aging. This seems most reasonable for cases with few or no NFT in the amygdala, hippocampus and nbM. This is also the neuropathology of pathological aging. Although it could be argued that pathological aging is pre-clinical AD, there is no a priori support for this hypothesis, and it also seems unlikely since it has not been possible to distinguish subjects with pathological aging from those with normal aging, even with prospective longitudinal evaluations (Delaere et al., 1990; Dickson et al., 1992). Were this truly a pre-clinical disease, it seems reasonable to expect to find change (i.e., decline) in at least some neuropsychological parameters.

On the other hand, some cases of DLBD are indistinguishable from AD, except for substantia nigra degeneration, Lewy body formation and CA2/3 neuritic degeneration. The SP in these cases have PHF-type neurites, and the neuropil also contains neuropil threads. Like AD, these cases also have many diffuse SP, but we would suggest that this form of SP may also reflect pathological aging in AD. These cases also have amyloid angiopathy in parenchymal and leptomeningeal vessels as frequently as do AD cases (Wu et al., 1992).

The increased frequency of AD in Lewy body disease has been frequently noted in the past (Gaspar and Gray, 1984; Jellinger, 1989; Gibb et al., 1989; Mastaglia et al., 1989); however, attention to the presence of cLB has not been possible until recently, with the development of ubiquitin-immunocytochemistry and monoclonal antibodies capable of distinguishing cLB from NFT. Furthermore, it is only recently that attention has been devoted to qualitative differences in SP in aging and AD (Dickson et al., 1988). It seems likely that some of the cases of combined AD and Parkinson's disease described in the literature reflect DLBD with co-existent pathological aging or AD.

In summary, the bulk of the current data suggests that, although amyloid deposition is common in DLBD, especially in those cases over the age of 60 years, it is not a necessary feature of DLBD. Furthermore, we do not believe that DLBD is a variant of AD, but rather that AD-type changes in DLBD represent co-existing conditions (pathological aging or AD).

References

Armstrong TP, Hansen LA, Salmon DP, Masliah E, Pay M, Kunin JM, Katzman R (1991) Rapidly progressive dementia in a patient with the Lewy body variant of Alzheimer's disease. Neurology 41:1178–1180

Ball MI, Hachinski V, Fox A, Kirshen AJ, Fishman M, Blume W, Kral VA, Fox H (1986) A new definition of Alzheimer's disease: a hippocampal dementia. Lancet 1:14–16

Bancher C, Lassmann H, Budka H, Jellinger K, Grundke-Iqbal I, Iqbal K, Wiche G, Seitelberger F, Wisniewski HM (1989) An antigenic profile of Lewy bodies: immunocyto-chemical indication for protein phosphorylation and ubiquitination. J Neuropathol Exp Neurol 48:81–93

Braak H, Braak E, Grundke-Iqbal I, Iqbal K (1986) Occurrence of neuropil threads in the senile human brain and in Alzheimer's disease: a third location of paired helical filaments outside of neurofibrillary tangles and neuritic plaques. Neurosci Lett 65:351–355

Burkhardt CR, Filley CM, Kleinschmidt-DeMasters BK, de la Monte S, Norenberg MD, Schneck SA (1988) Diffuse Lewy body disease and progressive dementia. Neurology 38:1520–1528

Byrne EJ, Lennox G, Lowe J, Godwin-Austen RB (1989) Diffuse Lewy body disease: clinical features in 15 cases. J Neurol Neurosurg Psychiat 52:709–717

Crystal H, Dickson D, Fuld P, Masur D, Scott R, Mehler M, Masdeu J, Kawas C, Aronson M, Wolfson L (1988) Clinico-pathologic studies in dementia: nondemented subjects with pathologically confirmed Alzheimer's disease. Neurology 38:1682–1687

Crystal H, Dickson DW, Lizardi JE, Davies P, Wolfson LI (1990) Antemortem diagnosis of diffuse Lewy body disease. Neurology 40:1523–1528

Davies P (1979) Neurotransmitter-related enzymes in senile dementia of the Alzheimer type. Brain Res 171:319–327

Davies L, Molska B, Hilbich C, Multhaup G, Martins R, Simms G, Beyreuther K, Masters CL (1988) A4 amyloid deposition and the diagnosis of Alzheimer's disease: prevalence in aged brains determined by immunocytochemistry compared with conventional neuropathologic techniques. Neurology 38:1688–1693

Delaere P, Duyckaerts C, Brion JP, Piette F, Hauw J-J (1989) Relationship between tau, paired helical filaments, amyloid and the intellectual deterioration in the neocortex in normal aging and in senile dementia of the Alzheimer type. In: Boller F, Katzman R, Rascol A, Signoret J-L, Christen Y (eds) Biological markers of Alzheimer's disease. Springer-Verlag, Berlin, pp 73–82

Delaere P, Duyckaerts C, Masters C, Beyreuther K, Piette F, Hauw J-J (1990) Large amounts of neocortical β/A4 deposits without neuritic plaques nor tangles in a psychometrically assessed, non-demented person. Neurosci Lett 116:87–93

Dickson DW (1990) Lewy body variant (correspondence). Neurology 40:486–493

Dickson DW, Yen S-H (1989) Beta-amyloid deposition and paired helical filament formation: Which histopathological feature is more significant in Alzheimer's disease? Neurobiol Aging 10:402–404

Dickson DW, Kres Y, Crowe A, Yen S-H (1985) Monoclonal antibodies to Alzheimer neurofibrillary tangles (ANT). 2. Demonstration of a common antigenic determinant between ANT and neurofibrillary degeneration in progressive supranuclear palsy. Am J Pathol 120:292–303

Dickson DW, Davies P, Mayeux R, Crystal HA, Thompson D, Goldman JE (1987) Diffuse Lewy body disease: neuropathological and biochemical studies of six patients. Acta Neuropathol (Berl) 75:8–15

Dickson DW, Farlo J, Davies P, Crystal HA, Fuld P, Yen S-H (1988) Alzheimer's disease: a double-labeling immunohistochemical study of senile plaques. Am J Pathol 132:86–101

Dickson DW, Crystal H, Mattiace LA, Kress Y, Schwagerl A, Davies P, Yen S-H (1989) Diffuse Lewy body disease: light and electron microscopic immunocytochemistry of senile plaques. Acta Neuropathol (Berl) 78:572–584

Dickson DW, Crystal HA, Yen S-H, Davies P (1990a) Alzheimer-Parkinson disease spectrum and diffuse Lewy body disease. In: Nagatsu T, Fisher A, Yoshida M (eds) Basic, clinical and therapeutic aspects of Alzheimer's and Parkinson's disease. Plenum Press, New York, pp 385–390

Dickson DW, Wertkin A, Kress Y, Ksiezak-Reding H, Yen S-H (1990b) Ubiquitin-immunoreactive structures in normal brains: distribution and developmental aspects. Lab Invest 63:87–99

Dickson DW, Wertkin A, Matiace LA, Fier E, Kress Y, Davies P, Yen S-H (1990c) Ubiquitin immunoelectron microscopy of dystrophic neurites in cerebellar senile plaques of Alzheimer's disease. Acta Neuropathol (Berl) 79:486–493

Dickson DW, Ruan D, Crystal H, Mark MH, Davies P, Kress Y, Yen S-H (1991) Hippocampal degeneration differentiates diffuse Lewy body disease (DLBD) from Alzheimer's disease: light and electron microscopic immunocytochemistry of CA2-3 neurites specific to DLBD. Neurology 41:1402–1409

Dickson DW, Crystal HA, Mattiace LA, Masur DM, Blau AD, Davies P, Yen S-H, Aronson MK (1992) Identification of normal and pathological aging in prospectively studied nondemented elderly humans. Neurobiol Aging 13:179–189

Finley D, Varshavsky (1985) The ubiquitin system: functions and mechanisms. Trends Biochem Sci 10:343–347

Forno LS (1986) The Lewy body in Parkinson's disease. In: Yahr MD, Bergmann KJ (eds) Parkinson's disease. Advances in neurology, vol 45. Raven Press, New York, pp 35–43

Galloway PG, Grundke-Iqbal I, Iqbal K, Perry G (1988) Lewy bodies contain epitopes both shared and distinct from Alzheimer neurofibrillary tangles. J Neuropathol Exp Neurol 47:654–663

Gaspar P, Gray F (1984) Dementia in idiopathic Parkinson's disease: a neuropathological study of 32 cases. Acta Neuropathol (Berl) 64:43–52

Ghanbari HA, Miller BE, Haigler HJ, Arato M, Bissette G, Davies P, Nemeroff CB, Perry EK, Perry R, Ravid R, Swaab DF, Whetsell WO, Zemlan FP (1990) Biochemical assay of Alzheimer's disease-associated protein(s) in human brain tissue: a clinical study. JAMA 263:2907–2910

Ghetti B, Tagliavini F, Masters CL, Beyreuther K, Giaccone G, Verga L, Farlow MR, Conneally PM, Dlouhy SR, Azzarelli B, Bugiani O (1991) Gerstman- Straussler-Scheinker disease. II Neurofibrillary tangles and plaques with Prp-amyloid coexist in an affected family. Neurology 39:1453–1461

Gibb WRG, Poewe WH (1986) The centenary of Friedrich H. Lewy. Neuropathol Appl Neurobiol 12:217–221

Gibb WRG, Esiri MM, Lees AJ (1987) Clinical and pathological features of diffuse cortical Lewy body disease (Lewy body dementia). Brain 110:1131–1153

Gibb WRG, Mountjoy CQ, Mann DMA, Lees AJ (1989) A pathological study of the association between Lewy body disease and Alzheimer's disease. J Neurol Neurosurg Psychiat 52:701–708

Glenner G (1979) Congophilic microangiopathy in the pathogenesis of Alzheimer's syndrome (presenile dementia). Med Hypotheses 5:1231–1236

Goate A, Chartier-Harlin MC, Mullan M, Brown J, Crawford F, Fidani L, Giuffra L, Haynes A, Irving N, James L, Mant R, Newton P, Rooke K, Roques P, Talbot C, Pericak-Vance M, Roses A, Williamson R, Rossor M, Owen M, Hardy J (1991) Segregation of a missense mutation in the amyloid precursor protein gene with familial Alzheimer's disease. Nature 349:704–706

Goldman JE, Yen S-H, Chiu F-C, Peress NS (1983) Lewy bodies of Parkinson's disease contain neurofilament antigens. Science 221:1082–1084

Guiroy DC, Liberski PP, Alwasiak J, Papierz, Gajdusek DC (1991) Demonstration of amyloid β-protein in a 32 year old man with progressive dementia. Acta Neuropathol (Berl) 82:523–526

Hansen L, Salmon D, Galasko D, Masliah E, Katzman R, DeTeresa R, Thal L, Pay MM, Hofstetter R, Klauber M, Rice V, Butters N, Alford M (1990) Lewy body variant of Alzheimer's disease: a clinical and pathological entity. Neurology 40:1–8

Hansen LA, Masliah E, Quijada-Fawcett S, Rexin D (1991) Entorhinal neurofibrillary tangles in Alzheimer disease with Lewy bodies. Neurosci Let 129:269–272

Hardy J, Allsop D (1991) Amyloid deposition as the central event in the aetiology of Alzheimer's disease. Trends Pharmacol Sci 12:383–388

Hirano A, Zimmermann HM (1962) Alzheimer neurofibrillary changes: a topographic study. Arch Neurol 7:227–247

Ince P, Irving D, MacArthur F, Perry RH (1991) Quantitative neuropathological study of Alzheimer-type pathology in the hippocampus: comparison of senile dementia of Alzheimer type, senile dementia of Lewy body type, Parkinson's disease and nondemented elderly control patients. J Neurol Sci 106:142–152

Jellinger K (1989) Pathology of Parkinson's syndrome. In: Calne DB (ed) Handbook of experimental pharmacology, vol 88. Springer-Verlag, Berlin, pp 47–112

Jellinger K, Danielczyk W, Fischer P, Gabriel E (1990) Clinicopathological analysis of dementia disorders in the elderly. J Neurol Sci 95:239–258

Katzman R, Terry RD, DeTeresa R, Brown T, Davies P, Fuld P, Reinbing X, Peck A (1988) Clinical, pathological and neurochemical changes in dementia: a subgroup with preserved mental status and numerous neocortical plaques. Ann Neurol 23:138–144

Katzman R, Aronson M, Fuld P, Kawas C, Brown T, Morgenstern H, Frishman W, Gidez L, Eder H, Ooi W-L (1989) Development of dementing illnesses in an 80-year-old volunteer cohort. Ann Neurol 25:317–324

Kawabata S, Higgins GA, Gordon JW (1991) Amyloid plaques, neurofibrillary tangles and neuronal loss in brains of transgenic mice over-expressing a C-terminal fragment of human amyloid precursor protein. Nature 354:476–478

Khachaturian ZS (1985) Diagnosis of Alzheimer's disease. Arch Neurol 42:109–1105

Kosaka K (1990) Diffuse Lewy body disease in Japan. J Neurol 237:197–204

Kosaka K, Yoshimura M, Ikeda K, Budka H (1984) Diffuse type of Lewy body disease: progressive dementia with abundant cortical Lewy bodies and senile changes of varying degree – a new disease? Clin Neuropathol 3:185–192

Kosaka K, Tsuchiya K, Yoshimura M (1988) Lewy body disease with and without dementia: A clinicopathologic study of 35 cases. Clin Neuropathol 7:299–305

Kure K, Lyman WD, Weidenheim KM, Dickson DW (1990) Cellular localization of an HIV-1 epitope in subacute AIDS encephalopathy using an improved double-labelling immunohistochemical method. Am J Pathol 136:1085–1092

Kuzuhara S, Mori H, Izumiyama N, Yoshimura M, Ihara Y (1988) Lewy bodies are ubiquitinated: a light and electron microscopic immunocytochemical study. Acta Neuropathol (Berl) 75:345–353

Lennox G, Lowe J, Morrell K, Landon M, Mayer RJ (1989) Anti-ubiquitin immunocytochemistry is more sensitive than conventional techniques in the detection of diffuse Lewy body disease. J Neurol Neurosurg Psychiat 52:67–71

Lennox G, Lowe JS, Godwin-Austen RB, Landon M, Mayer RJ (1989) Diffuse Lewy body disease: an important differential diagnosis in dementia with extrapyramidal features. In: Iqbal K, Wisniewski HM (eds) Proceedings of the first international conference on Alzheimer's disease and related disorders. Alan R. Liss, New York, pp 121–130

Lowe J, Blanchard A, Morrell K (1988) Ubiquitin is a common factor in intermediate filament inclusion bodies of diverse type in man, including those of Parkinson's disease, Pick's disease and Alzheimer's disease, as well as Rosenthal fibers in cerebellar astrocytomas, cytoplasmic bodies in muscle and Mallory bodies in alcoholic liver disease. J Pathol 155:9–15

Mann DMA, Jones D (1990) Deposition of amyloid (A4) protein within the brains of persons with dementing disorders other than Alzheimer's disease and Down's syndrome. Neurosci Lett 109:68–75

Mark MH, Sage JI, Dickson DW, Schwartz KO, Duvoisin RC (1992) Levodopa non-responsive Lewy body parkinsonism: clinicopathologic study of two cases. Neurology 42, in press

Masliah E, Terry RD, Mallory M, Alford M, Hanse LA (1990) Diffuse plaques do not accentuate synapse loss in Alzheimer's disease. Am J Pathol 137:1293–1297

Mastaglia FL, Masters CL, Beyreuther K, Kakulas BA (1989) Deposition of Alzheimer's disease amyloid (A4) protein in the cerebral cortex in Parkinson's disease. In: Iqbal K, Wisniewski HM (eds) Proceedings of the first international conference on Alzheimer's disease and related disorders. Alan R. Liss, New York, pp 475–484

McKee A, Kosik K, Kowall NW (1991) Neuritic pathology and dementia in Alzheimer's disease. Ann Neurol 30:156–165

Pappolla MA (1986) Lewy bodies of Parkinson's disease: immune electron microscopic demonstration of neurofilament antigens in constituent filaments. Arch Pathol Lab Med 110:1160–1163

Pericak-Vance MA, Haines JL, St George-Hyslop PH, Bebout J, Haynes C, Tanzi R, Yamaoka L, Gusella JF, Roses AD (1991) Collaborative linkage analysis of chromosome 19 and 21 loci in familial Alzheimer's disease. Soc Neurosci Abstr 17:195

Perry EK, Marshall E, Perry RH, Irving D, Smith CJ, Blessed G, Fairbairn AF (1990) Cholinergic and dopaminergic activities in senile dementia of Lewy body type. Alzheimer Dis Assoc Disorders 4:87–95

Perry RH, Irving D, Blessed G, Fairbairn A, Perry EK (1990) Senile dementia of the Lewy body type: A clinically and neuropathologically distinct form of Lewy body dementia in the elderly. J Neurol Sci 95:119–139

Reisert I, Pilgrim C (1991) Sexual differentiation of monoaminergic neurons – genetic or epigenetic? Trends Neurosci 14:468–473

Richardson RT, DeLong MR (1988) A reappraisal of the functions of the nucleus basalis of Meynert. Trends Neurol Sci 6:264–267

Roberts GW, Allsop D, Bruton C (1990) The occult aftermath of boxing. J Neurol Neurosurg Psychiat 53:373–378

Roberts GW, Gentleman SM, Lynch A, Graham DI (1992) β/A4 amyloid protein deposition in brain after head trauma. Lancet 338:1422–1423

Robertson M (1992) Alzheimer's disease and amyloid. Nature 336:103

Roses AD, Gilbert JR, Bartlett RJ, Pericak-Vance MA, Dawson DV, Morrison MR (1987) Sib-pair linkage and subtraction analysis of familial Alzheimer's disease. In: Davies P, Finch CE (eds) Molecular neuropathology of aging, Banbury report, vol 27. Cold Spring Harbor Laboratory, New York, pp 443–456

Schellenberg GD, Bird TD, Wijsman EM, Moore DK, Boehnke M, Bryant EM, Lampe TH, Nochlin D, Sumi SM, Deeb SS, Beyreuther K, Martin GM (1988) Absence of linkage of chromosome 21q21 markers to familial Alzheimer's disease. Science 24:1507–1509

Schmidt ML, Murray J, Lee V M-Y, Hill WD, Wertkin A, Trojanowski JQ (1991) Epitope map of neurofilament protein domains in cortical and peripheral nervous system Lewy bodies. Am J Pathol 139:53–65

Schwartz P (1970) Amyloidosis. Cause and manifestation of senile deterioration. Charles C Thomas Publ, Springfield, IL

Selkoe DJ, Bell DS, Podlisny MB, Price DL, Cork LC (1987) Conservation of brain amyloid proteins in aged mammals and humans with Alzheimer's disease. Science 235:873–877

St George-Hyslop PH, Haines JL. Farrer LA, Polinsky R, Van Broeckhoven C, Goate A, Crapper McLachlan DR, Orr H, Bruni AC, Sorbi S, Rainero I, Foncin JF, Pollen D, Cantu J-M, Tupler R, Voskresenskaya N, Mayeux R, Growdon J, Fried VA, Myers RH, Nee L, Backhovens H, Martin J-J, Rossor M, Owen MJ, Mullan M, Percy ME, Karlinsky K, Rich S, Heston L, Montesi M, Mortilla M, Nacmias N, Gusella JF (1990) Genetic linkage studies suggest that Alzheimer's disease is not a single homogeneous disorder. Nature 347:194–197

Tanzi RE, Gusella JF, Watkin PC, Bruas GAP, St George-Hyslop P, Van Keuren ML, Patterson D, Pagan S, Kurmit DN, Neve RI (1988) Amyloid β-protein gene: cDNA, mRNA distribution and genetic linkage near the Alzheimer locus. Science 235:880–884

Terry RD, Masliah E, Salmon D, Butters N, DeTeresa R, Hill R, Hansen L, Katzman R (1991) Physical basis of cognitive alterations in Alzheimer's disease: synapse loss is the major correlate of cognitive impairment. Ann Neurol 30:572–580

Tomlinson BE (1989) Second Dorothy S. Russell Memorial Lecture: The neuropathology of Alzheimer's disease – issues in need of resolution. Neuropathol Appl Neurobiol 15:491–512

Tomlinson BE, Blessed G, Roth M (1968) Observations on the brains of nondemented old people. J Neurol Sci 7:331–356

Wisniewski T, Haltia M, Ghiso J, Frangione B (1991) Lewy bodies are immunoreactive with antibodies to gelsolin related amyloid-Finnish type. Am J Pathol 138:1077–1083

Wolozin BL, Pruchnicki A, Dickson DW, Davies P (1986) A neuronal antigen in the brains of Alzheimer patients. Science 232:648–650

Wu E, Lipton RG, Dickson DW (1992) Amyloid angiopathy in diffuse Lewy body disease. Neurology 42, in press

Yen S-H, Dickson DW, Crowe A, Butler M, Shelanski ML (1987) Alzheimer's neurofibrillary tangles contain unique epitopes and epitopes in common with the heat-stable microtubule associated proteins tau and MAP2. Am J Pathol 126:81–91

Yoshimura N, Yoshimura I, Asada M, Hayashi S, Fukushima Y, Kudo H (1988) Juvenile Parkinson's disease with widespread Lewy bodies in the brain. Acta Neuropathol (Berl) 77:213–218

Subject Index